Daniel Langford, DMin, MSW
Emil J. Authelet, DMin

When the Caregiver Becomes the Patient
A Journey from a Mental Disorder to Recovery and Compassionate Insight

Pre-publication
REVIEWS,
COMMENTARIES,
EVALUATIONS . . .

"**A**ll therapy is essentially biography, a life story told by those who experience healing and hope through spiritual caregiving as a secular sacrament. When the man who was born blind received his sight through the caring touch of Jesus, his healing became his biography: `One thing I do know, that though I was blind, now I see' (John 9:25). When clients emerge from the darkness of their pain with a story of healing to tell, we know that the caregiver is a good therapist. When the therapist tells his or her own story of recovery and healing, as Dan Langford has done in this remarkable book see that caregiving can also be a m sacrament of spiritual healing. W

in the form of a conversational dialogue with his own therapist, Emil Authelet, *When the Caregiver Becomes the Patient* both informs and edifies. Armed with clinical insight, seasoned with spiritual wisdom, and permeated with unpretentious self-disclosure, Langford and Authelet tell their story, which is, of course, the story of all who dare to be caregivers and those who seek their care. This book is a must-read for the journey."

Ray S. Anderson, PhD
Professor of Theology and Ministry,
῾ical Seminary,

"**A** fine and unique perspective on caregiver as mental health patient, and the process and meaning of recovery. Langford and Authelet find meaning and opportunity in the crisis of mental illness, and the rich complexity of the issues facing family members and those who seek to provide care and support. Critical, well-focused attention is given to the role of Christian spirituality in healing, as well as the empowering strength that may be shared by the giver and recipient of care. Rarely are we offered such a powerful book that offers a profoundly moving description of what it feels like to be in the middle of a mental breakdown and a difficult recovery process, and a broad-ranging discussion of what the experience has meant (and might mean) to all those who have been part of it. Langford and Authelet's work stands as a challenge to a narrow medical view of caregiving in the twenty-first century."

Professor John L. Erlich
Division of Social Work,
California State University,
Sacramento

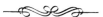

"**I**n *When the Caregiver Becomes the Patient: A Journey from a Mental Disorder to Recovery and Compassionate Insight,* Daniel Langford, with a collaborating friend and professional colleague, takes the reader through the spiritual odyssey of self-discovery that led him to a more nearly complete human authenticity. He does this by recounting the practicalities and vicissitudes of living related to a near collapse of his personal functioning and to the path for securing help. His themes are that all persons are vulnerable and that the personal self and the professional self are inseparable.

From the very beginning of the book, his lucidity of writing, clarity of expression, and exposition of feeling are compelling and revealing of his profound humanity. His insightful analysis and critique of research on the features of mental disorder (including physiological, psychological, and sociocultural dimensions), adds an invaluable examination of the spiritual aspects of behavior and of treatment approaches. The book is very rich in content and utilizes system theory, phenomenology, existential themes, and humanist concepts to provide depth and meaning to his experience and journey. Transactional analysis is applied to his experience for even greater depth. All of this leads Dr. Langford to conclude that a caregiver is an agent of healing who aids and stands beside the person being served. Two chapters are devoted to how the caregiver's personal suffering benefits clients, and this is done with clear and useful enumeration of caregiver characteristics. The authors each provide new models pertaining to the caregiver-client relationship and, through dialogue, present a new vision of therapy."

Juan D. Hernández, MSW
Professor Emeritus,
Division of Social Work,
California State University,
Sacramento

When the Caregiver Becomes the Patient

A Journey from a Mental Disorder to Recovery and Compassionate Insight

THE HAWORTH PASTORAL PRESS
Religion and Mental Health
Harold G. Koenig, MD
Senior Editor

When the Caregiver Becomes the Patient

A Journey from a Mental Disorder to Recovery and Compassionate Insight

Daniel Langford, DMin, MSW
Emil J. Authelet, DMin

The Haworth Pastoral Press®
An Imprint of The Haworth Press, Inc.
New York • London • Oxford

Published by

The Haworth Pastoral Press®, an imprint of The Haworth Press, Inc., 10 Alice Street, Binghamton, NY 13904-1580.

Cover design by Anastasia Litwak.

Excerpt from THE SEVEN STOREY MOUNTAIN by Thomas Merton, copyright 1948 by Harcourt, Inc. and renewed 1976 by the Trustees of The Merton Legacy Trust. Reprinted with permission of the publisher.

Material from Agras, W. S. (1985). *Panic: Facing Fears, Phobias, and Anxiety* reprinted with permission of W. H. Freeman and Company.

Excerpts from *Fully Human, Fully Alive* by John Powell, S. J. © 1976 John Powell, S. J. Resources for Christian Living, Allen, TX 75002. Reprinted with permission of the publisher.

Excerpts from ON BECOMING A PERSON by Carl Rogers. Copyright © 1961 by Carl R. Rogers. Reprinted with permission of Houghton Mifflin Company. All rights reserved.

Library of Congress Cataloging-in-Publication Data

Langford, Daniel L.
    When the caregiver becomes the patient : a journey from a mental disorder to recovery and compassionate insight / Daniel L. Langford, Emil J. Authelet.
        p. cm.
    Includes bibliographical references and index.
    ISBN 0-7890-1293-6 (alk. paper) — ISBN 0-7890-1294-4 (alk. paper)
    1. Caregivers—Case studies. 2. Care of the sick—Psychological aspects. I. Authelet, Emil.
II. Title.

R727.47 .L364 2002
362'.0425—dc21

2001051589

CONTENTS

ABOUT THE AUTHORS

Daniel L. Langford, DMin, MSW, received his Doctor of Ministry from Fuller Theological Seminary in 1994, and his Master of Social Work from California State University, Sacramento, in 1996. He has more than 30 years experience as a health care professional, teacher, social worker, and pastoral minister. He is the author of *The Pastor's Family: The Challenges of Family Life and Pastoral Responsibilities* (Haworth).

Dr. Emil J. Authelet, DMin, MDiv, has more than 30 years experience as a pastoral minister and consultant to pastors and churches in crisis.

Foreword

It is a common myth that caregivers, whether they are pastors, psychologists, psychiatrists, or counselors, never experience any significant emotional disorders. After all, they are trained to recognize the symptoms and to help others who suffer from these problems, not become victims themselves. The truth is that caregivers are human also. They are subject to the same stress, the same interpersonal tensions, and the same genetic influences as everyone else. It is true that some troubled people may become caregivers themselves as a way of solving their own personal problems. They will be particularly vulnerable. Most caregivers who succumb are no different from anyone else—they are just ordinary people.

It may surprise others when a caregiver experiences an emotional disturbance, but no one is more surprised than the caregivers themselves. Their defenses are supposed to be impenetrable. They are trained to recognize the early signs of trouble, and they should have all the skills for survival already in tow. When emotional problems do strike, caregivers fear that they may be doubly defective—defective in their own makeup and defective in the application of what they should know.

This book is a personal account of the struggle confronting a caregiver who suffers a serious emotional disruption—a panic anxiety disorder. Dan Langford is as candid and sincere as anyone can be. His account of how the attacks began, their precursors, and his journey toward wholeness is both illuminating and encouraging for other caregivers. His road to recovery was driven by a determination to find out as much as he possibly could about this disorder. The fruits of his discoveries are presented in clear, nontechnical language that both enlightens and encourages those who might follow in his footsteps.

The disorder to which Dan succumbed is by no means uncommon. Panic anxiety disorder is now the number one mental health problem for women in the United States. It is second only to substance abuse in men, many of whom may well be "self-medicating" through alcohol or drug abuse. One report from the National Institute of Mental Health says that thirty-five percent of young adults have reported at least one panic attack in the previous year. By my observation, the problem continues to show a steady increase in incidence.

The consequences of panic disorder can be quite debilitating, as Dan so clearly describes. Panic attacks can strike without warning and can be about the most frightening experience anyone can imagine. They seldom strike the "weak," but by their nature seek out the strong and driven. The reason is not hard to discern since it is stress that is the primary causal mechanism, and those who live a hurried and hassled lifestyle are at greatest risk.

If there is one valuable lesson that sufferers from panic disorder can learn, it is that what they are experiencing is not their fault. They are certainly not going crazy. I say this because so many of my own panic attack patients have somehow come to believe that they either have a weak personality or they simply lack the inner strength to deal with the circumstances of their lives. Worse still, some even believe that they suffer because their mother didn't love them enough or because they committed the "unpardonable sin." In reality, the brain is just doing what it is designed to do when it sets up the conditions for panic. It is sending warning signals that we are pushing ourselves beyond the limits of our unique design.

Another valuable lesson the reader can take from this book is that the future looks very bright for those who suffer from panic and anxiety disorders. New medications and psychotherapy treatment strategies have been developed that can prevent a patient from becoming dependent on their medication and ensure long-term success without forcing the sufferer to severely restrict his or her activities. Right now at least 90 percent of sufferers can expect to find effective relief. Nothing can top such good news!

Archibald D. Hart, PhD, FPPR
Professor of Psychology and Dean Emeritus
Graduate School of Psychology
Fuller Theological Seminary;
Author of The Anxiety Cure

Preface

From the conception of this story to its birth, the United States and the world have gone through bipolar epochs that have left us all (like Tevye in *Fiddler on the Roof*) staring bewilderingly heavenward with open palms and grief-stricken countenances, just asking for understanding. As happened to Tevye, the wedding (our sense of peace and safety) has been destroyed, and we want to know why.

In the summer of 1999, when this story of my panic attacks began, the pendulum of life had swung to the pole of prosperity. Our nation and the whole world were in the midst of the dot-com boom. The ethereal prosperity of this boom appeared to be never-ending. Notwithstanding those good times, the emperors created by the dot-com boom did not know that their tailors were frauds. The naked emperors shocked their stockholders and themselves when they watched their castles in cyberspace come tumbling down midway through the first year of the millennium. The new economy lacked substance. So, by the end of 2000, the pendulum of life swung to the opposite pole, and the dot-com boom became the dot-com bust.

The year 2001 arrived, and we as a nation struggled to clean up the economic mess. By the end of the summer, we appeared to be making progress with the repair of the economy. Then, when we thought hope was dawning once more, two planes crashed through that dawn on September 11, 2001, and instantly we all became like Rachel, "weeping for our children" and other loved ones (see Matthew 2:18). In shock, we beheld the carnage and mourned beside the rubble that was once the World Trade Center. We grieved (all of us) in a cloud of choking, gray dust that rained deluges of office memos and business contracts that were once a part of enterprises that vanished in a ball of exploding jet fuel. The only sounds around us besides our sobs and the patter of tears hitting the gray dust were the cricketlike stridulations of alarms on downed firemen that painfully chirped the news that our rescuers did not make it either. What a bewildering world!

These were the events that occurred after *When the Caregiver Becomes the Patient* was written. Consequently, as one of the authors of this book, I have been haunted by this question: "Where does my story about recovery from panic fit into a world of people who have suffered far more than I could ever imagine suffering?" Here are some of the answers I stumbled upon.

First, as my co-author Emil Authelet observed, "All of us as human beings experience personal 'ground zeros' somewhere and sometime in our life journeys." The tragedy of the World Trade Center is a colossal reflection of the innumerable "ground zeros" experienced by human beings everywhere, all the time. "Ground zero" may be as intense as a death, or it may be a seemingly insignificant panic attack. Nevertheless, all such events come crashing into our lives at unexpected moments, and we stand before them helplessly trying to understand the tribulations that have befallen us. The "ground zeros" we corporately experience include such things as aging, terminal illness, divorce, financial ruin, the death of loved ones, and shattered dreams. No human is insulated from adversity, and this is the first way I discovered that my story connects to our bipolar world.

The second answer to my question has to do with friends. "Ground zeros" are inexplicable, but friends during such times are indispensable. My story is a story about friends. Emil and David were my rescuers. They were survivors who came alongside and helped me through the devastation of my meltdown by offering the comfort and support I so desperately needed.

The next three answers were surprisingly revealed in the last verse of the Apostle Paul's "hymn of love" found in 1 Corinthians: "And now faith, hope, and love abide, these three; and the greatest of these is love" (1 Corinthians 13:13, RSV).

Hence, the third answer is about faith. My experience with panic attacks is a story about the reestablishment of faith. Arndt and Gingrich (1979) stated that one translation of the Greek word *pistis* (faith) is a "belief and trust in the Lord's help in physical and spiritual distress" (p. 663). My belief and trust in God have taken on new and deeper meanings as a result of a painful journey through panic.

The fourth answer is about hope. The Greek *elpis* (hope) can be translated as "expectation" (Arndt and Gingrich, 1979, p. 253). For me, hope was the anticipation and expectation of recovery. Emil, in the midst of my crisis with panic, said to me, "Dan, this will not last.

You will get better." Thus, my friend gave me hope. We all want hope that "ground zeros" do not last forever.

Finally, the fifth answer is about love. Arndt and Gingrich (1979) stated that *agape* (a Greek term for love) specifically refers to human love in 1 Corinthians 13:13 (p. 5). This *agape* is the highest expression of human virtue that is orchestrated by God. I experienced this *agape* from my friends, and their choice to love gave me the courage to believe and hope anew.

Accordingly, *When the Caregiver Becomes the Patient* connects to these universals of human experience:

1. Our personal worlds explode and come apart unexpectedly.
2. Providentially, in the midst of the chaos, we discover we are not alone.
3. We find friends who come alongside us and rekindle our hope and faith.
4. But most important, the friends we discover in our darkest hours show what love really is when the chips are down and life seems hopeless.

This is the story you are about to read.

Dan Langford

Chapter 1

A Frightening Summer Experience

Daniel Langford

Hot and Horrid August Nights

August 1999, was not the best of times for me. I had a frightening experience that gave new meaning to the passages in the Psalms that talk about darkness and the "slimy pit" as associated with hopelessness and death. My experience was what clinicians call "free-floating anxiety," which was coupled with a panic attack that lasted for more than a month.

I suppose the most frightening thing about this experience was that my brain, which I and most of us take for granted, began to do some crazy things. Through this experience, I felt as though I had lost control of the functions of my mind and was a helpless bystander while rumination, irrational fear, and panic took over the normal functioning of my brain.

Further unsettling was that I was not prepared for the impact of this malady, despite my training and disparate professional roles as a pastor, social worker, and schoolteacher.

Precursors to the Meltdown

When I reflect upon the months and days that preceded the August meltdown, I realize I might have been more prepared for what I was about to experience had I been paying attention.

My wife, Diana, and I had been through a pressure cooker of stressors, and my assumption was that if I could just "hang in there" and keep fighting, these stressors could be conquered. What I failed to understand was that the pressures of life exact a dear price on our emotions and resiliency. Further, if the number and intensity of stressors become too great, such pressures can cause a breakdown in one's ability to cope, and the weakest parts of one's being begin to malfunction.

This happened to me. Here is a short history of the events that pre-dated the summer of 1999.

An Unexpected Move and Changes of Employment

Through circumstances beyond either my or Diana's control, we felt compelled to leave careers that we had shared for over eight years at a nursing home in Northern California. Diana worked as the Director of Nursing Services, and I was the social worker at this facility.

Because of matters of mismanagement and improprieties on the part of the owner/administrator, we felt we could no longer serve in this location and, as a result, tendered our resignations on July 31, 1998.

What followed was two months of job searches and the pressures of relocation. We traveled over 10,000 miles during August and September, chasing down numerous leads and experiencing the frequent disappointments that come with starting over. Our search ended in the small town of Lakeport, California, where Diana accepted a new position as Director of Nurses at another nursing home.

Diana's job fell into place first, but I continued my job search, hoping to find a social work position that would allow me to begin earning hours toward certification as a licensed clinical social worker.

What resulted, instead, was an offer to teach language arts and social studies at Oak Hill Middle School in Clearlake, California. The confidence placed in me by the principal, as well as a generous salary package, prompted me to return to an eighth-grade classroom, which was how my varied career had begun more than thirty-four years earlier. Concurrently, this turn of events intrigued me because my career journey had become a circle rather than a straight line. Hence, the phrase "What goes around comes around" has taken on a new meaning for me.

Despite the blessings of this new job, plenty of trouble came with the new position. Oak Hill Middle School serves a population of students who are challenged by severe problems with poverty, domestic violence, and substance abuse in their homes and community. For these reasons, teaching in this setting is very difficult.

Further, the classes I took over in October 1998 had gone through five substitutes since the beginning of the school year, and the students were unruly and angry. In fact, this upset was severe enough to spawn a committee of students and parents who appeared before the school board demanding that they be given a regular teacher. I was selected as that "regular teacher," but I never became a messiah. Consequently, what followed was weeks and months of agonizing effort to turn around the negative forces affecting these unhappy students and to create a positive learning environment.

This change did not come quickly and easily, because the anger and upset of the students persisted. One reason for the unhappy emotions expressed by the students may have been grief over the loss of a favorite teacher who had taken a job at the high school shortly after the school term began and whose departure created the vacancy that I was filling.

Hence, between October 1998 and April 1999, I was engaged in a war with an unhappy cohort of middle-school students as well as unhappy parents. I took an extra week off during the spring break and seriously considered not returning because of the stress and the daily battle of wills that had to be waged with these students. Nonetheless, I decided to finish the school year and, to my grateful surprise, the overall mood of the students changed for the better. The classes became more manageable and cooperative, so that I was able to finish the year with modest success.

Despite the positive changes, the stress tied to this job took its toll on both my physical and emotional well-being. As a result, the pressures of this teaching experience, coupled with the life-changing stressors that preceded it, became the incubator of the physical and emotional meltdown I was about to experience.

The Summer of 1999

School was over, and the summer of 1999 began uneventfully. Nonetheless, both Diana and I continued to deal with the adjustments that came with our relocation.

Most important, we had left behind a beautiful home in our previous locale that was surrounded by an acre of redwood trees. We sacrificed this home for a small apartment with no yard. In addition, our belongings remained in storage, and our efforts to buy another home had been fruitless. Hence, uncertainty over and dissatisfaction with our living conditions further eroded my emotional resiliency. The pressures I felt were about to reach a climax.

The Final Straw That Precipitated the Meltdown

During July, before the fateful meltdown of August 1999, I took a temporary summer job as a social worker at a nursing home in a community near my school. I soon discovered that this job created even more pressure, because the resident population of this facility had a significant number of people who were experiencing high anxiety. Consequently, with the stressors I was already experiencing, this was not the best of working environments. I also wonder if we caregivers are more susceptible and vulnerable than others to the spiritual and emotional states of the people for whom we provide care.

Again, I assumed that I could handle anything. "After all," I said to myself, "I am a strong, masculine individual; it is just a matter of willpower and hanging in there."

As the weeks progressed and the challenges escalated in this nursing home, I realized that just "hanging in there" was not working. The residents' problems started to become overwhelming. I began to overidentify with the circumstances of many of these individuals, and the salve of detachment, which allows so many in the medical profession to be able to serve patients with difficult diagnoses, began to wear thin. I was taking the weight of the world on my shoulders. The accumulation of previous stressors was breaking down my coping abilities. A collapse was imminent.

The Onset of Panic

The first manifestations of this physical, cognitive, and emotional crisis occurred during morning meetings at the nursing home where I was working. When the morning report was given, staff members were crowded into a small room with one door and no windows. The cramped space, coupled with the oppressive August heat, exacerbated the problems I already had with discomfort in closed-in places. The cramped setting for these meetings became intolerable, especially when the sessions were long. I made it a point to sit by the door, but this did not always help, particularly when the air-conditioning did not function properly. I began to dread going to work.

Further manifestations of this meltdown developed over the next few weeks during early morning hours at home. One regular and frightening experience was waking up at 2:00 a.m. with the perception that an indescribably negative force was dragging both me and my mind into a pit of darkness from which there was no escape. These dark thoughts made no sense and had no substance. I had the feeling that the oppressive force was dragging me down, and I felt helpless to control this force or my thoughts about it. When this oppression was at its peak, I would get up in these "dead of the night" hours and walk the streets, trying to shake the gloom. I kept saying to myself, "This is crazy. I cannot pin my thoughts down. My brain is out of control, and the negative oppression I am feeling is more than I can bear." The experience was terrifying.

In addition to the negative power that had taken over my thinking (and that occurred at the same time every night), I experienced an increase of claustrophobic terror. For a number of days, I could not even sleep in the bedroom of our apartment. I set up a cot outside in the carport, or I placed the cot by the open front door of our apartment. In addition, I had no tolerance for darkness. The room I was sleeping in had to be flooded with light. All of this seemed so irrational. I felt as if I was standing outside of my mind watching helplessly while my brain produced ruminations, irrational fear, and panic that I could not control.

I soon discovered that the placement of my cot in sites of escape to alleviate terrifying thoughts provided only a temporary respite. In a short time, irrational and negative thoughts kicked in regardless of where I tried to sleep. It was at this point that I felt despairingly trapped in a vortex of tormented thinking patterns from which there was no escape. I fantasized that I would not physically be able to bear the torture that my out-of-control brain was inflicting upon my body. I was losing hope.

A Ground Crew of Rescuers

Two rescuers were part of the ground crew that talked my out-of-control mind out of this near-fatal tailspin to a safe landing that re-established my ability to perform routine daily activities without the irrational fear I was experiencing. My wife led me to the first rescuer.

Diana, who is an RN, was very patient throughout this ordeal. She had never seen me in quite the state I had tumbled into, but she was aware that there might be a medical cause for the troubles. Interestingly, Diana was under the same, if not more, pressure that I was, but she did not go through the meltdown I experienced.

Diana suggested that I contact David Betat, who was the medical director of her nursing home and had recently become our family doctor. I phoned Dr. Betat's office with a complaint of free-floating anxiety, and an appointment was scheduled immediately.

I didn't tell Dr. Betat until later, but my first appointment with him only exacerbated my terror. I did everything I could to keep my panic under control when I arrived at his office. First, his waiting room was crowded with people, and it was dark. Second, there was only one door in and out of the office, which was frequently blocked by his patients. It took all the willpower I had not to bolt for that door and/or move the people out of the way.

I was directed into one of his patient rooms. Again, this was a dimly lighted, very small space with the windows covered by thick curtains. Dr. Betat came in, sat on his examining stool, and positioned himself between me and the closed door of the room. Deep inside, I screamed silently in terror while I maintained an outward appearance of calm. During this time, I kept assuring myself that the ordeal would be over in a few minutes, then I would be free again.

When I talked about this experience with Dr. Betat later (or rather when my wife talked to him, since I was somewhat embarrassed), he was deeply apologetic for what had happened. He explained to Diana and to me later that his first concern was confidentiality, so he had closed the door to ensure privacy. He would not have placed me in that examining room had he known what effect it was having upon me.

Notwithstanding this anxious beginning, Dr. Betat became a copilot who guided me with compassionate care out of the darkness I was experiencing.

Dr. Betat told me this:

> Dan, you are not crazy. You are experiencing chemical imbalances in your brain that are causing these thoughts. In addition, your family history as you have described it may carry a gene that is causing the claustrophobia. Finally, by your own statement, you recognize that you are predisposed to compulsive behavior, which again is likely to be hereditary. Therefore, the mix

of the above conditions, which have been further affected by environmental stressors, has likely created the situation you are experiencing today. Again, you are not crazy. This is a medical problem.

Dr. Betat communicated a biospiritual understanding of my situation that provided great comfort and relief. In addition, Dr. Betat prescribed a very low dose of BuSpar, which over time took the panicky edge off my thoughts and appeared to calm and stabilize the functioning of my brain.

A second rescuer, Dr. Emil Authelet, completed the rescue with a psychosociospiritual perspective.

Emil and I have known each other for more than nine years. He was my regional supervisor when I served as a pastor for the American Baptist Churches of the West. Through the years that I have worked with him, Emil has become a friend, mentor, and confidant.

When I called Emil and described my experiences to him, he connected with me almost immediately in spirit and in deep understanding. He was able to reflect back almost instantly the exact circumstances of my plight. I was surprised that he knew so much about what I was going through when I had given him only a very sketchy introduction.

Emil got right to the point:

> Dan, I believe that your experience with panic is only temporary, but what you are going through belies deeper issues way down inside of you that are being expressed through the panic attacks. Yes, you are an adult who has lived almost fifty-seven years. You function well, and you have achieved many goals and obtained an advanced education. Nevertheless, as I see it, there is a child inside of you who is running: a child who still has not resolved the issues of his past. You still fail to see yourself as God sees you, which is as a person who is worthy to be loved. The child in you does not believe he is worthy of love.

We continued the discussion as Emil explored this obscure and suppressed part of my being, and he encouraged me to consider that one aspect of healing the panic attacks was to come to a new understanding of my personal worth as a person when all the masks, achievements, and status are stripped away. When life is torn back to that frightened little boy huddled in a dark corner of the adult soul, Emil said, "that little boy that is you needs a healing understanding of who he is. He is a worthwhile and valuable human being who has every right to love and be loved in return."

I can describe only in a limited way the stirring I began to feel deep within the core of my being as I talked to Emil over the next few weeks. It was hard to come to terms with the reality that we can live for a considerable time with darkness and unresolved issues which, when they surface at critical times, provide a deeper understanding of who it is that we identify as our real selves. Emil said, "You need an overhaul in your thinking so that you might really know what it means to love who you are. The boy need not run any longer."

Emil subsequently recommended that I read John Powell's book, *Fully Human, Fully Alive: A New Life Through a New Vision.* John Powell believes, through his own experiences and through the insights he gained from others on human perception, that misconceptions distort our understanding of who we are and the reaction we have to the world around us. Hence, panic attacks such as the ones I experienced have not only an organic root (imbalanced brain chemistry) but also can be connected to our psychospiritual selves. Powell (1976) observes the following:

> As we have said previously, all negative emotions, but especially anxiety and hostility, are signals of a malignant misconception somewhere in our total vision. We cannot afford to pass over such reactions with a comment that we will feel better tomorrow. . . . All negative feelings, from the mildest discomfort to the deepest depression, will lead us to a moment of insight if only we will follow. (p. 115)

A Journey of Discovery and Healing

Consequently, this book will be my story of exploration, discovery, and healing. My encounter with panic attacks not only reminded me of my vulnerability but also that "life continues to ask me questions," as John Powell so eloquently puts it.

Emil Authelet will accompany me as co-author as we embark on this journey. Our purpose is quite simple. All of us as human beings struggle with life somewhere and sometime. Regardless of who we become or what we achieve, the common thread we share as members of the human family is our fragility in an often difficult world. No one is immune or invincible.

Moreover, the professional who provides physical and emotional healing to others is effective in his or her craft only if such a professional recognizes his or her vulnerability to the same struggles the patients experience. To paraphrase Thomas Merton, all of us have darkness in our lives; we share in some measure the good and evil of all humanity. Our effectiveness as healers increases when we discover those dark places and find the light that leads us to greater maturity and integration of ourselves. The lessons we learn will comfort and heal those we are called to serve.

Chapter 2

Critique of the Literature
on Panic Attacks

Daniel Langford

INTRODUCTION

A Personal Touch

As will be evident by the number of references provided in this book on the origin and etiology of panic attacks, an abundant base of literature has been created by doctors and other experts in this field who are far more qualified than I am to analyze and discuss this phenomenon. Rather than add to the extant literature on panic attacks, I will attempt to interpret and apply such research to my own experience, which will be qualified by the interview with Dr. Betat in Chapter 3, who was the primary clinician who assisted in my rescue.

We See Through a Glass Darkly

This critique of the literature will attempt to address my experience with panic attacks from a holistic perspective, which was not always the approach taken by researchers. My wife, Diana (who is an RN and has observed over the past thirty years numerous cycles in the field of medicine regarding strategies for treatment), contends that the current approach to providing therapy for a medical problem may be in vogue because of the marketing pressure of a certain drug company trying to promote a new drug and/or because of the political climate in the medical establishment at the time certain approaches and medications are the "medicus receptus."

Author von Bertalanffy (1974) argues in a similar fashion that culture and politics influence what is accepted as truth even in the so-called exact sciences. Here is his position as to why deterministic "robot psychology" was proselytized in the first half of the twentieth century:

> American psychology in the first half of the twentieth century was dominated by the concept of the reactive organism, or more dramtically, by the concept of the model of man as a robot. . . .
>
> The tenets of robot psychology have been extensively criticized in the works by Allport, Matson, Koestler, von Bertalanffy, and others. The theory, nevertheless, remained dominant for obvious reasons. The concept of man as a robot was both an expression of and a powerful motive force in industrialized mass society. It was the basis for behavioral engineering in commercial, economic, political, and other advertising and propaganda; the expanding economy of the "affluent society" could not subsist without such manipulation. Only by manipulating humans ever more into Skinnerian rats, robots, buying automata, homeostatically adjusted conformers and opportunists (or bluntly speaking, into morons and zombies) can the great society follow its progress toward an ever increasing gross national product. As a matter of fact, the principles of academic psychology were identical with those of the "pecuniary conception of man." (p. 1996)

Consequently, despite a researcher's attempt to be objective with double-blind experiments or whatever approach is chosen, there does not appear to be a single or pure path to resolving psychological or medical problems, simply because the human element is present at all times and is influenced by politics, culture, and the prevailing worldviews. To illustrate this point, if we lived in a society that rejected the scientific method and looked to the ministrations of witch doctors as the answer for medical/mental problems, not only would our methods be different, as influenced by politics and culture, but the accepted outcomes would also be a product of such a different political/cultural climate.

With reference to this idea, William Hendricks (1980) asserted that contemporary Western culture sees the world with multiple lenses of past worldviews. According to Hendricks, our Western culture first inherited a Greek worldview, which attempts to describe phenomena. Second, Western culture is influenced by the Roman worldview, which attempts to take things apart to see how they work. This Roman influence is no doubt the foundation for research based on the scientific method. Finally, because of the impact of Judaism via its offspring, Christianity, Western culture is influenced by a "hear, see, and obey" response to phenomena in a Hebraic faith statement that declares, according to Hendricks, "God is known by what he does" (pp. 63-65).

Hence, our worldview and/or the mix of worldviews certainly influences outcomes and assertions. So, despite our attempts as human beings to create pure science, data, or faith, such ideals do not exist. Our attempts to explain reality are shots in the dark; purity in any discipline is elusive.

All of these things considered, I will attempt to interpret my experience with panic attacks through the eyes of researchers in the fields of medicine, psychology, and social phenomena with the recognition that we see darkly through the glass of truth.

A PANIC ATTACK AS DEFINED BY THE DSM-IV

The *Diagnostic and Statistical Manual of Mental Disorders* (DSM-IV) (American Psychiatric Association, 1994) is the principal clinical reference used by health professionals in multiple disciplines to define and diagnose mental disorders. The DSM-IV defines a panic attack as follows:

> A **Panic Attack** is a discrete period in which there is the sudden onset of intense apprehension, fearfulness, or terror, often associated with feelings of impending doom. During these attacks, symptoms such as shortness of breath, palpitations, chest pain or discomfort, choking or smothering sensations, and fear of "going crazy" or losing control are present. (p. 393)

The DSM-IV goes on to list the criteria for a panic attack with these qualifiers: a discrete (distinct or separate) period of intense fear or discomfort along with four or more of the following symptoms, which develop abruptly and reach a peak within ten minutes:

1. palpitations, pounding heart, or accelerated heart rate
2. sweating
3. trembling or shaking

4. sensations of shortness of breath or smothering
5. feeling of choking
6. chest pain or discomfort
7. nausea or abdominal distress
8. feeling dizzy, unsteady, lightheaded, or faint
9. derealization (feelings of unreality) or depersonalization (being detached from oneself)
10. fear of losing control or going crazy
11. fear of dying
12. paresthesias (numbness or tingling sensations)
13. chills or hot flushes (p. 395)

Finally, the DSM-IV indicates that panic attacks can occur spontaneously ("out of the blue"), or they can be situationally cued (i.e., connected to an anticipated, stressful event) (pp. 394-395).

The DSM-IV and My Experience

When I reflect on the panic I experienced, the apparent DSM-IV symptoms were numbers 9 and 10. I unquestionably experienced being detached (standing outside my body observing this crazy ordeal) and felt as if I were going crazy. However, I did not experience any somatic symptoms other than the adrenaline rush when I would wake out of sleep at 2:00 a.m. I did not sweat, have heart palpitations, or experience the feeling that I was going to die. I was just damned uncomfortable and really felt I had lost control of my brain and its functioning.

In addition, these intense feelings and the accompanying meltdown appeared to be linked to the situational stressors, which included our forced move and problems controlling the behavior of students at my teaching job. I also remember that when the stressors decreased, the feelings of panic were significantly reduced, and I eventually quit taking prescribed medication (BuSpar) since I felt it was no longer necessary. Consequently, the following things come to mind when I consider the DSM-IV criteria for a panic attack and my experience.

First, the benchmark for a DSM-IV diagnosis hinges on the impairment of normal life functioning related to a specific event. In addition, a diagnosis for a panic attack must include four of the thirteen symptoms previously mentioned. Considering these criteria, my experience with panic did not reach the level described in the DSM-IV. I only experienced two of the four symptoms, and, except for the loss of sleep during the early morning hours, I carried on a normal schedule of work. Furthermore, the DSM-IV notes, "A panic attack is not a codable disorder" (p. 395).*

All of these factors considered, here is my point. I believe the DSM-IV describes life crises that are universal to everyone. The difference between a clinical diagnosis in the DSM-IV and common human experience includes multiple symptoms and the intensity of a disorder, which disrupts the normal life functioning of the patient. Consequently, whether patient or therapist, maladies occur in individual cognitive and emotional responses to life stressors that are universal in one way or another to every man and woman. Human vulnerability is universal. Furthermore, the difference between universal human experience and clinical frailty is the degree of disablement, the intensity and life-disrupting effect of a mental/emotional problem as modeled in the DSM-IV. From my perspective, the border that separates the so-called normal state from a disability is ethereal.

Here are some illustrations. Everyone gets the blues, but do your blues affect the quality of your life and interfere with the normal routines of living? Fear of heights is a common fear for many people, but does this fear dissuade you from following the normal course of daily events and keep you from entering tall buildings or traveling on steep mountain roads?

Hence, the caregiver in one way or another is connected to the vulnerability of his or her patient/client. The caregiver shares similar, if not the same, fears and struggles with his or her patient, but the caregiver's fears and struggles are usually not disabling nor do they interfere with the routines of life.

Other Opinions on the DSM-IV Taxonomy

As I stated previously, I did not feel as though I experienced four or more of the symptoms of a panic attack. The DSM-IV defines panic attacks with fewer than four symptoms as "limited-symptom attacks" (p. 394).

---

*Quoted material in this section has been reprinted with permission from the *Diagnostic and Statistical Manual of Mental Disorders*, Fourth Edition. Copyright 1994 American Psychiatric Association.

In light of the strict criteria for a panic attack diagnosis in the DSM-IV, Norton, Pidlubny, and Norton (1999) cited David Barlow and others, and recommended a conservative assessment of non-clinical panic attacks (those not under the care of a physician). In a significant part of their discussion, the authors argue that some events labeled as panic attacks may simply be experiences of intense emotions related to the effects of a stressor. They comment as follows:

> When evaluating the aspects of panic or panic attacks, it is highly recommended that investigators be very conservative in their definition of nonclinical panic attacks. Based on Norton et al. (1992) and more recent studies that have attempted to better define nonclinical panic (Brown and Deagle, 1992; Cox et al., 1994; Hayward et al., 1997; Wilson et al., 1992), the following recommendations are provided for defining nonclinical panic attacks. First, consistent with the findings of Brown and Deagle (1992), the definition of a panic attack should be detailed and specifically exclude attacks that occur during actual physical threat. . . . Second, the time frame used for assessing panic attacks should be reduced from one year to three months to reduce memory distortions. . . . Third, based on the findings of Cox et al. (1994), people who report only one attack in the 3-month period should not be classified as NPAs unless they present evidence of panic-related distress. Forth [sic], a panic attack should be defined as having at least four symptoms that are at least moderately severe. Finally, if it is difficult in questionnaire-based studies to determine if self-reported panic attacks occurred during actual threat situations, then the person should report distress or impairment (e.g. avoidance) as a result of the panic attacks. (p. 327)*

THE MATRIX OF PANIC ATTACKS

Stewart Agras (1985) approached the problem of panic disorders from a holistic perspective. Based on his discussion, I will look at the

*Norton, R., Pidlubny, S. R., and Norton, P. J. (1999). Prediction of panic attacks and related variables. *Behavior Therapy*, 30, 319-330. Copyright 1999 by the Association for Advancement of Behavior Therapy. Reprinted with permission of the publisher.

various precipitators of panic attacks and then relate them to my own experience.

Biological Factors

Physiology and Neurochemistry

Consistent with his expertise as a physician, Agras discusses chemical reactions and other phenomena that occur between our old brain and our new brain.

The old brain, according to Dr. Agras, includes a region known as the septo-hippocampal region (p. 59). The new brain, or cerebral cortex, sits above this region. According to Agras, the septo-hippocampal region of the brain acts as a comparator, "matching incoming information about the environment, which is processed in the cerebral cortex" (new brain) (p. 59). Agras declares further that if the events processed by the cerebral cortex "match up," then the septo-hippocampal region operates in a checking mode. However, if a mismatch occurs, Agras states that the septo-hippocampal region takes control of ongoing behavior and inhibits it (p. 59).

Agras goes on to describe an experiment with a sea snail called an Aplysia. The snail eats only seaweed, but it can recognize chemicals given off by the juice of a shrimp. In the experiment with the Aplysia, an electric shock was sent to the sea snail's head when shrimp juice was present. The combination of shock and the presence of shrimp juice created an avoidance reaction in the snail that Agras described as a miniphobia. Agras contends that the Aplysia experiment may show that nerve cells change in form and respond to neurotransmitters based on the experience of the organism (pp. 60-61).

Weiss and Uhde (1990) discuss the same experiment, which was conducted by Kandel (1983). The researchers concluded that changes occurred in the sensory neurons and interneurons related to the reactions to neurotransmitters which would heighten an avoidance reaction in the sea snail when aversive stimuli were present.

If the Aplysia experiment mirrors molecular changes that may occur in the human nervous system, I can understand, by my own experience, how a continued bombardment of stress and negative experiences could change the way the brain and nervous system respond to such forces. The "old brain," which regulates physiological functioning of the body, compares messages from the "new brain," where the cognitive activity occurs, in order to determine whether the organism will fight or flee a given situation. Concurrently, if chemical sensitivity to anxiety-provoking neurotransmitters also increases in the brain and nervous system as a result of the interaction between the cognitive interpretation of events and the primal survival mechanisms of fight or flight, I understand how the whole neurochemical circuitry of the brain and the respondent body can malfunction to the point of creating those out-of-control feelings I experienced. I can honestly say that I felt I had no control over what was going on in my brain or how my body was reacting.

Agras (1985) concludes his discussion with these observations:

> Learning interacts with biology within the cells of the nervous system. One likely point of interaction, as we have seen from research with the sea snail, is at the end of a sensory neuron. Here, avoidance learning results in an increase in the number of active zones at which a neurotransmitter is released. It seems likely that a similar mechanism takes place in humans. The release of neurotransmitters in avoidance learning may well affect the benzodiazepine receptor site, which in turn affects the setting of the comparator mechanism in the old brain, either diminishing or increasing avoidance behavior. (p. 64)

Inheritance and Anxiety

Closely allied to all of the above is the possibility that inheritance may play a part in predisposing some people to increased fearfulness. Agras (1985) considers two components of inheritability when it comes to predispositions to anxiety. One component, he said, is molded by our link to our primal ancestors, and the other is the newer concept of a genetic predisposition to stress based on family inheritance. First, we will consider the ancient biological links that Agras asserts we have with primal man and animals.

Primal fears. Agras contends that three categories of fears exist: fears of animals, of injury, and of separation from others (p. 32). Agras traces these fears back in time to the primeval function of survival. Agras argues:

> We are living in the bodies of our ancestors, bodies shaped by centuries of existence in a harsh environment quite different

from that of modern times. The brisk response to a sudden noise or to a visual cue suggesting the form and movement of a reptile, while still useful today, was a necessity for survival in times past. The rapid response to such events . . . is a complex integrated behavior undoubtedly shaped by its success in preserving life through countless generations. Even though we no longer live in such a physically dangerous world, these automatic reactions live on in our bodies. (p. 23)

Agras discusses how basic human fears occur in the animal kingdom as well. Human infants as well as primate infants appear to have an inbuilt "nursemaid of fear" that kicks in as the young child or primate becomes separated from its mother (p. 30). Hence, fear is a survival mechanism that protects the young human or primate from danger or harm as it grows.

Translating the origin and purpose of primal fears as tools of survival in a hostile environment and the protection of the very young, Agras connects common phobias to these primordial origins. In a study of a sample of residents living in Burlington, Vermont, the most common fears included fears of snakes, heights, storms, injury, enclosed places, and being alone. These fears are linked to the basic fears just described: fears of animals, injury, and separation. Consequently, although we do not live in the harsh and primitive environment of our ancestors and animal counterparts, the fears that protected these ancestors and animals persist in modern life and in our adult experience. These are fears that should disappear as we grow into adults. Yet, for complex reasons, these fears often persist.

In addition, Agras makes an interesting connection to the primal past and fears in females. In a study he conducted which has been corroborated by other researchers, he found that women tend to express more fears than men do. Although social conditioning that allows women greater freedom to express feelings of fear may be a reason women report more fear than men report, Agras argues again for a more primal origin. He states that women are less physically able to defend themselves in the wild and also need extra protection during childbirth. "This may be nature's way of ensuring the survival of humanity. Thus the propensity for women in our society to have more fears than men may have both biologic and social roots" (p. 33). In summary, Agras suspects that a relationship exists between basic fears and phobias (p. 34).

Family heredity. A second element of the biological origins of phobias, anxiety, and panic is the possible connection to a genetic inheritance from either side of a family of origin.

Crowe (1990), in his article on molecular genetics, notes that in a collection of data from twelve studies spanning over fifty years (based on family history interviews with patients) evidence exists that neurocirculatory asthenia (weakness) appears to run in families and corresponds to reports of patients with panic disorder (pp. 63-64). The most significant correlations are with patients who report that first-degree relatives (parents and siblings) are to some degree affected by neurocirculatory asthenia and panic disorder. It is interesting to note that Crowe documents females experience panic disorder at two or three times the rate of males, which is concurrent with information provided by Agras and previously discussed in this chapter.

Crowe goes on to discuss the linkage between the results of genetic marker studies and panic disorder. Crowe states that research with a group of twenty-nine markers so far has not confirmed a statistically significant link to panic disorder (p. 66). Hence, the ability to separate nature from nurture in determining the causes of phobia, panic, and anxiety remains elusive.

In tandem, Agras (1985) may be on the right track when he argues that learning and heredity may be very difficult to separate. Agras contends that learning and heredity are inextricably tied together (p. 37). Those doing research on the subject of anxiety and panic should consider a dual rather than an either/or distinction regarding the origins of anxiety and panic.

Twin studies. Some of the most significant research must be done with twins, according to Agras. Since 1985, when Agras published his book on panic, I have found two reports on twin studies that attempted to determine a significant family link to panic disorders.

The first was a report by Torgersen (1990). In his conclusion, he states that genetic factors "seem" to be involved in the incidence of panic disorders with monozygotic twins. "However," Torgersen states, "most MZ twin pairs are discordant, pointing to the importance of environmental factors" (p. 56). Again, this substantiates the complicated link between learning/environment and heredity as discussed by Agras.

A more recent study on twins was reported by Stein, Jang, and Livesley (1999). Although the researchers reported a strong heritable component of anxiety sensitivity among monozygotic twins, the results again were not conclusive that genetics alone contributed to the problem of anxiety, phobias, and panic (pp. 246-251).

Therefore, current research on panic and anxiety may be seriously erring by taking a reductionist stance on the origins of panic disorder. Von Bertalanffy (1974) stated in his principles of social theory that the whole of human existence is greater than the sum of its parts ("non-summativity") (p. 1111).

No easy answers. In retrospect, the matrix of human experience related to the causes of panic and anxiety includes biology, brain chemistry, animal behavior, heredity, genetics, learning, and environment. In addition, a spiritual dimension exists which is the primary focus of this book. Hence, the components of this matrix do not fit neatly into a double-blind experiment. We, as humans, are more than the results of a laboratory experiment.

Brain Chemicals and Neurotransmitters

This subject was mentioned in the discussion of the physiology of the brain and how the nervous system may be affected at a molecular level by interactions of our cerebral response ("new brain"), to life stressors and the septo-hippocampus ("old brain"), which controls body responses through the autonomic nervous system. Research is currently underway to determine if chemical imbalances in the brain and nervous system may cause a predisposition to panic attacks.

Artificially provoked panic attacks. Griez and Schruers (1998) documented two experiments in which panic was induced in volunteers by introducing substances into the body which created a panic attack. The first of these substances was part of an experiment initiated by Pitts and McClure (1967). Sodium lactate was administered to fourteen anxiety-prone individuals and ten healthy controls. The self-report of thirteen of fourteen of the anxiety-prone individuals stated they experienced symptoms of a panic attack following the infusion. However, only two of the ten controls responded with distress to the sodium lactate infusion (Griez and Schruers, 1998, p. 495).

A second substance used to induce an artificial panic attack was carbon dioxide. In an experiment by Gorman and colleagues (1987), it was again found that those individuals predisposed to anxiety reported symptoms of a panic attack when given a 35 percent inhalation of carbon dioxide. The same experiment reported that members of the control group who inhaled the CO_2 experienced some "neuro-vegetative symptomatology resembling that of a panic attack," but none of the controls stated they experienced anxiety (Griez and Schruers, 1998, p. 497).

Related to these laboratory-induced panic attacks, Medscape (2000) commented on laboratory-provoked panic attacks with cautious words about the experiments. First, the writers noted that critics of provocation studies argue that the evidence "for a biological etiology of PD (panic disorder)" is inconclusive (p. 2). Second, when sodium lactate was given to volunteers to provoke panic, only the patients with a history of panic disorder responded with fear to the physiological sensations brought on by the sodium lactate introduced into their bodies.

Similarly, Griez and Schruers (1998) acknowledge that although the "experimental pathophysiology of panic has produced an impressive body of literature," an instructive hypothesis is still lacking (pp. 500-501).

Benzodiazepine pathways and brain chemistry. Agras (1985) discusses how brain-mapping research with benzodiazepines (anti-anxiety/antidepressant drugs) has provided new information on the electrochemical reactions in the brain and nervous system that may be linked to panic attacks.

Agras states, "In 1977, two research groups reported the existence of specific receptor sites in the brain with an affinity for benzodiazepines" (p. 58). At these sites there appeared to be three docking areas. One was for the benzodiazepine molecule. A second was for endogenous (internal) compounds that caused anxiety in animals. Finally, a third docking area was used by substances that block both the effects of benzodiazepines and anxiety-provoking compounds. Agras suggested that the identification of these receptor sites presupposes that substances are secreted by the brain which induce fear/anxiety, while the brain also secretes other substances that block the fear/anxiety reaction. Agras states, "Their precise ratio may lead either to the emotionally stable or to the nervous individual" (p. 58).

Thus, Agras effectively argues a case for chemical reactions in the brain that may influence a person's response to stressors which have the potential to create panic. Agras's discussion of the brain's reaction to chemicals and its own secretions connects to my feeling of helplessness when I felt my brain was out of my control during a panic attack. I remember that I imagined I was standing outside my body and saying to myself, "Something is wrong here. My brain is doing crazy things, and I have no power to control what is going on." Thus, it appears to be possible, if Agras is right, that substances (chemicals) in my brain which induce panic were inadequately counterbalanced by those substances in the brain which alleviate panic.

Sapolsky and the biology of depression. Before we leave the biological arena, I want to consider briefly the perspectives of Sapolsky (1994) on the biology of depression, who closely parallels the arguments presented by Agras on brain-chemical homeostasis.

Numerous studies on panic disorder propose that a link exists between panic and depression (Klerman et al., 1993, p. 27). Hence, factors related to the development of depression may be similarly related to the experience of panic.

With this in mind, Sapolsky (1994) proposes that stress creates biological changes in the brain that lead to depression. Significant in this discussion is Sapolsky's exposition of the "pleasure pathway" hypothesis.

Sapolsky cited research done several years ago by neuroscientists who discovered that the human brain has a pleasure pathway. That is, if certain parts of the brain are stimulated with electrodes, the person experiences significant feelings of satisfaction, pleasure, and well-being. Sapolsky states that indications suggest that synapses along this pleasure pathway use the substances norepinephrine and serotonin. Sapolsky goes into considerable detail explaining the various hypotheses as to how depression develops in the superabundance or lack of these chemicals in the pleasure pathway and other parts of the nervous system (pp. 206-210). The significance of Sapolsky's discussion is its concurrence with Agras's "new brain-old brain" interactions.

Sapolsky maintains that negative thoughts can create reactions in the parts of the brain below the cerebral cortex that can cause the body to react as if it had been "gored by an elephant." Here is what he says:

> Now what happens during a depression? You think a thought—about your mortality or that of a loved one; you imagine children in refugee camps; rainforests disappearing and endless species of life evaporating; late Beethoven string quartets—and suddenly you experience some of the same symptoms as after being gored by an elephant. On an incredibly simplistic level, you can think of depression as occurring when your cortex thinks an abstract neg-

ative thought and manages to convince the rest of the brain that this is as real as a physical stressor. In this view, people with chronic depressions are those whose cortex habitually whispers sad things to the rest of the brain. (pp. 211-212)

The power of thoughts. What is the result of all this? Signals of danger are sent to parts of the brain that control bodily reactions. Chemicals in the nervous system get out of balance; the body reacts to a stressor in an exaggerated way; and panic, anxiety, or depression kick in. Plato might be right after all: Ideas are a powerful force, and the mind really can make the body sick.

Given these considerations, the power of negative thoughts to create negative bodily reactions builds a case for the restructuring of our thinking. The restructuring of our thoughts, which encompasses who we think we are and our perception of life experiences, appears to be an effective route to healing the mind and body from the effects of life events and stressors. This restructuring of thought (particularly in the spiritual dimension) is a major theme of this book. Concurrently, cognitive-behavioral therapy, which involves at least in part a change in thought patterns, is considered one of the most effective treatments of panic disorder apart from drug therapy (American Psychological Association, 2000, pp. 4-6). Further, Klerman et al. (1993) offer evidence that pharmacological therapy combined with psychological interventions such as cognitive-behavioral therapy may be the best of treatments (pp. 103-108). This concurs with Agras's contention that learning and biology are interconnected and are quite difficult to separate when considering the phenomenon of panic (pp. 133-134).

Psychological Theories That May Explain Causes of Panic Attacks

Psychodynamic Theories

Agras (1985), who is the benchmark for our exploration of panic and panic attacks, retells a 1909 case history by Sigmund Freud titled "The Analysis of Phobia in a Five-Year-Old Boy" (p. 41). The boy had a fear of horses that Freud attributed to the boy's sexual desire to have his mother to himself. Agras comments as follows on Freud's interpretation:

As a result of Freud's advice, a long series of conversations between Hans and his father began, in which various sexual longings were discussed. These conversations, duly reported in 140 pages, led to the basic interpretation of the phobia, namely, that Hans wanted to have his mother to himself but was afraid that his father would retaliate. Thus, he displaced his fear of being injured (castrated?) by his father onto the horse, which, like his father, had a big widdler, and which threatened to bite him. A big fear hid behind a little fear! Moreover, by avoiding horses and staying at home, he gained more attention from his mother, thus achieving one of his aims. Such economy is, in Freud's view, one of the hallmarks of neurosis. (p. 42)

Agras notes that critics of Freud's approach argue that any number of interpretations are possible in this scenario. Furthermore, conversations between Hans and his father may have influenced consequent behavior and given rise to a self-fulfilling prophecy (p. 43).

Other researchers who discuss psychodynamic theories of panic attacks are Klerman et al. (1993). These commentators noted, as did Agras, that psychodynamic theory attributes some forms of panic apprehension as "the emergence of deeply rooted unconscious conflicts, primarily aggressive in character, that originated in traumatic experiences in early childhood" (p. 42).

Nonetheless, Medscape (2000) contends, as do Agras (1985) and Klerman et al. (1993), that psychodynamic assertions lack research data. The writers of the Medscape article stated that, "although psychodynamic formulations are interesting," some of these formulations are based on "unconscious etiologies" which are, "difficult to test directly and even more difficult to refute" (p. 4).

The Cognitive Model and Causes of Panic Attacks

A second category of psychological rationale for the causes of panic attacks and panic disorder involves a misinterpretation of events and/or exaggeration of the danger that may be connected to these events. Hence, phobias, reactions to somatic phenomena such as a rapid heartbeat, and exaggerated reactions to routine life events can trigger panic (Medscape, 2000; Barlow and Bufka, 1999; Klerman et al., 1993).

Treatment from the cognitive-behavioral perspective (discussed later) includes helping the sufferer to reframe thoughts as well as providing gradual exposure to a feared experience (such as looking down from a tall building) to reduce and eventually eliminate the panic that comes from being placed in such a stressful circumstance.

Social Factors, Life Events, and the Relationship to Panic and Panic Attacks

Systems Theory and the Analogy of a Mobile

A teaching colleague of mine and former social worker commented perceptively about the impact of life events on families. Cognizant of systems theory, my colleague reflected as follows:

> When we work with a child in the classroom, we are working with the systems in that child's life, be they family, peers, or community. Those systems are connected just like a mobile. You touch one system or one part of the mobile, and the whole mobile or interconnection of systems is set in motion. (Maes, 2000)

Maes summarizes the essence of a holistic approach in understanding the phenomena of human behavior. Von Bertalanffy (1974), who was cited earlier in this chapter, proposes that all human beings are connected to systems which interact in complex ways in any person's life. Understanding human behavior as emanating out of a matrix of systems interacting one with the other, be they family, community, job, nation, religion, friendships, or even the physical body itself, could lead researchers to a more inclusive discernment of the nature and causes of panic attacks. Hence, the examination of social factors in determining the etiology of anxiety, depression, and panic disorders shows that we as human beings are more than the physiology of our brains or the functioning of our minds.

The Positive and Negative Effects of Family Systems on the Recovery from Panic Disorders

Agras (1985) addresses both the positive and negative influences of systems in relation to panic. The example he uses is the family system, which can be a valuable arena of support for an individual struggling with issues related to panic. However, such a family system can also be destructive and hinder the healing of a person with a panic problem.

Agras addresses the tendency of a family system to keep a balance or homeostasis within itself, which has the potential of hindering the recovery of a member experiencing panic. Family-system homeostasis occurs when a family unit becomes adjusted to the illness of the afflicted member and consequently resists making changes necessary for that person's recovery or healing. If a condition such as panic or depression remains unchanged, then the system continues to be in balance because the family has adjusted to the member's problems. If the afflicted person gets better, then the balance is upset and, notwithstanding the prior suffering of the afflicted member, the family system is thrown into crisis because other family members must change to adapt to the improvement of the recovering member. Agras explains it this way:

> . . . If something changes in one part of the system, the entire system is perturbed, and an offsetting change must occur in other areas to reestablish balance.
>
> Such a theory suggests that a symptom such as agoraphobia would tend to be maintained so that other family members could remain unperturbed, fixed in their accustomed roles. Should an agoraphobic begin to improve, then one of several changes would be set in motion: Adaptive behavior might occur on the part of other family members; another family member might develop symptoms; or failing such adjustments, the marriage might break up. (p. 110)

Multiple System Breakdowns: Tales of Panic and Loss of Control

In contrast to a family system hindering the healing of a panic victim because of its predisposition to maintaining homeostasis, the multiple systems in a person's life can create panic, anxiety, and a sense of loss of control when crises and traumatic events disrupt the functioning of those systems.

I have had frequent opportunities to share my experiences of panic with acquaintances and extended family members. I discovered that many of them shared almost identical experiences of panic. Significantly, in every case, the panic was connected to a stressful life event. Here are some of the stories:

Bill. Bill described what it was like to go through a divorce. He remembered the stress of the divorce "put his brain into overload" and panic kicked in. His symptoms were very much like mine. He saw a counselor and had to take time off from work.

Jane. Jane and her husband experienced financial loss and the foreclosure of a home. Following these traumatic events, Jane told me that for the longest time she could not stay inside her home at night. She felt the walls closing in, and she walked the streets as I did in the early morning hours, plagued with anxiety and insomnia.

Travis. Travis had his life threatened by gang members. Since this distressing occurrence, Travis has experienced such post-traumatic stress reactions as free-floating panic and hypervigilance.

Diana. This final story is my wife's experience. Diana lost her mother to congestive heart failure a few weeks before this book was completed. Although she has not experienced full-blown panic in her grief, Diana describes an intolerance for low ceilings and cramped living situations. As she puts it, "I want to push up the ceilings and move the walls away."

All of the aforementioned situations show that social factors related to life events (and our perception of those events) can lead to panic.

Klerman et al. (1993) address the phenomena of life events as precipitants of panic:

> Many studies indicate that significant life events precede the onset of panic disorder (Faravelli, 1985; Last et al., 1984; Roy-Byrne et al., 1986).
> . . . Faravelli (1985), with a more systematic approach, found a higher number of life events in patients with a first panic attack compared with healthy control subjects in the twelve months preceding the onset of panic attacks, noting that "both loss events and threatening events seem to play a role" (p. 105) in the onset of panic anxiety. In addition, Roy-Byrne and colleagues (1986) found that panic patients reported significantly more life events in the 12 months preceding their first panic attack compared with control subjects. The patients also reported significantly more subjective distress about their life events compared with control subjects, and events were viewed by the patients in comparison

with the control subjects as more undesirable and uncontrollable and having caused extreme lowering of self-esteem. (Klerman et al., 1993, pp. 53-54)

UNDERSTANDING PANIC
USING AN INTEGRATED MODEL

Multidetermined Causal Models

Concurrent to this discussion, Barlow (1992), like Agras (1985), argues for "multidetermined causal models." Barlow believes that "linear causal models will give way to multidetermined causal models," when researchers look for the causes of panic disorders (p. 2). His assertion is that both psychological and biological factors contribute to the creation of panic. He goes on to say that drug therapy paired with psychological interventions may be an effective treatment for panic.

In a similar way, Agras (1985) states that understanding the causes and treatment of panic necessarily integrates biology with learning:

> We have seen that the once separate approaches of biology and learning now merge at two levels—in certain processes in the brain cell, where learning seems to affect chemical control systems; and in external behavior, where the combination of drugs and exposure therapy has proven most effective in treating the agoraphobic with panic. An understanding of the interaction between learning and biology is essential to the further unraveling of both the cause and cure of phobias and panic. (p. 133)

Nevertheless, despite the affirmations of Agras and Barlow for integration of biology and learning as an eclectic path to understanding panic, they do not go far enough. Two essential ingredients for understanding have been left out of the model. Maybe the problem is that the missing two ingredients do not always pack well into a scientific investigation. The missing ingredients are the social factors (distinct from psychology) and the spiritual factors.

These last two elements are critical for an understanding of the totality of the human experience. Human beings are more than biology; human beings are more than conditioned learning. Human beings are also social; human beings become who they become because of the people they meet, the surroundings they live in, and the experiences they go through. Finally, human beings are spiritual; who human beings are and become is ultimately related to a human being's connection to God. A human being's relationship to God is the capstone for a complete holistic experience of life, and this capstone as it relates to my experience with panic will be the focus of my story.

TREATMENTS FOR PANIC

The concluding section in this exploration of the literature on panic attacks examines treatment approaches. I have attempted to connect the book's approaches with the current literature on panic.

Pharmacological Treatment

Buspirone

My experience with buspirone. During the height of my crisis with panic, I received a prescription for buspirone, which has the trade name of BuSpar. When Dr. Betat gave me this medication, he stated that I would have to be patient in waiting for results. The drug was not fast acting and would take about two to three weeks before beginning to decrease the anxiety I was experiencing. Part of the reason for graduated doses is that the side effects of immediate, full use of the drug, which include dizziness, have discouraged some from continuing with the treatment.

Nonetheless, I remember that the three weeks waiting for the BuSpar to take effect were maddening. The symptoms of anxiety were at their peak, and I remember being emotionally exhausted from the effects. I wanted instant relief. Despite this angst, I followed the regimen for the dosages and, ultimately, the therapy contributed to my healing.

The two things I appreciated about using BuSpar were that it did not become habit forming and the one side effect I felt (which was occasional lightheadedness) was not that objectionable. Ultimately, when my life experiences became less stressful, when brain chemicals became more balanced, and when my worldview was once again centered on hope and serenity, I discontinued the BuSpar therapy, intuitively understanding that the medication was no longer necessary—and I was correct.

Nevertheless, the BuSpar treatment was very important for my recovery. I am very thankful that the medication was available, and I am grateful to the physician who provided the treatment.

A short history of buspirone. Cadieux (1996) states that buspirone is part of a class of drugs called azapirones. Buspirone was the first of this class of drugs introduced in 1986.

According to Cadieux, azapirones are effective in treating anxiety in a way similar to the benzodiazepines but without the "sedative, muscle relaxant or anticonvulsant properties"; in addition, the azapirones do not appear to be habit forming (p. 1).

Interestingly, Cadieux maintains that the drug is not effective for a panic attack or other forms of crisis intervention because the drug takes at least two weeks to become effective, and no euphoric feeling accompanies its use (p. 2).

My physician recommended buspirone more for the long-term resolution of anxiety rather than for treating the panic attacks. Because I was very resistant to taking any medication at all, the choice of buspirone was excellent: the drug had minimal side effects and it treated long-term problems, such as intrusive thinking and rumination (Cadieux, 1996, p. 3).

How buspirone might work. Both the *Nursing 95 Drug Handbook* (1995) and the Gale Group (2000) indicate that how buspirone functions to relieve symptoms of anxiety is really not known. The best guess is that buspirone decreases both the amount and actions of a chemical called serotonin in specific parts of the brain (Gale Group, 2000, p. 1).

Serotonin, according to Moeller (1999), is a chemical that is produced in the brain from the amino acid tryptophan. Moeller acknowledges that researchers still do not understand the complete function of serotonin, but an imbalance of the chemical in certain parts of the brain can contribute to such psychiatric disorders as depression and obsessive-compulsive disorder with accompanying repetitive and disturbing thoughts.

Benzodiazepines

A family of drugs that has been around longer than the azapirones are the benzodiazepines.

In an interview with Mark H. Pollack, the *Harvard Mental Health Letter* ("What Are the Current," 2000) noted that benzodiazepines such as alprazolam (Xanax) and clonazepam (Klonopin) are used to treat panic disorder because they are fast acting. Nonetheless, the article noted such side effects as drowsiness, dizziness, intellectual impairment, and the risk of physical dependence.

Agras (1985) summarizes the effects of benzodiazepines in his discussion of the "new brain" (cognition) interacting with the "old brain" (autonomic response), which we explored earlier in this chapter. The brain has receptor sites for benzodiazepines. The introduction of benzodiazepines at these receptor cites leads to the secretion of gamma-aminobutyric acid, or GABA. This chemical blunts the "old brain's" comparator reactions and disrupts the inevitable somatic reactions that would come about with distressing emotional thoughts from the cerebral cortex. Hence, benzodiazepines put the fight-or-flight mechanism on hold through the introduction of the chemical GABA.

Tricyclic Antidepressants

A third group of antianxiety drugs are the tricylics, which are so named because of their biochemical structure (Sapolsky, 1994, p. 205). Two commonly used tricylics to treat anxiety are imiprimine (Tofranil) and clomipramine (Anafranil). The *Harvard Mental Health Letter* ("What Are the Current," 2000) indicates that the primary purpose of these tricylics is to treat depression. However, they are also effective in the treatment of panic disorders (p. 2).

Sapolsky (1994) states that tricylics work to relieve depression by allowing the neurotransmitter norepinephrine to remain in the synapse longer. When this reuptake of norepinephrine is slowed, the neurotransmitter is likely to hit its receptors a second or third time. Sapolsky goes on to say that the presence of norepinephrine stimulates the sympathetic nervous system, and the subsequent decrease in depressive symptoms allows the increased functioning of the pleasure pathways in the brain (pp. 205-207).

Nonetheless, as with the benzodiazepines, the *Harvard Mental Health Letter* ("What Are the Current," 2000) states that serious side effects come with the use of tricylics. Some of these side effects include "dry mouth, blurred vision, a rapid heartbeat, lightheadedness, and weight gain" (p. 2).

Serotonin Reuptake Inhibitors

A fourth group of drugs are known as selective serotonin reuptake inhibitors (SSRIs). These drugs include paroxetine (Paxil), sertraline (Zoloft), fluoxetine (Prozac), citalopram (Celexa), and fluvoxamine (Luvox). I noted in the discussion on buspirone that balancing serotonin in certain parts of the brain helps to relieve anxiety. SSRIs are drugs of choice for treating panic attacks because of their immediate effectiveness ("What Are the Current," 2000, p. 2). Side effects include nausea, drowsiness, and decreased sexual functioning (*Nursing 95 Drug Handbook,* 1995, pp. 410-411).

Monoamine Oxidase Inhibitors

A fifth class of drugs that is effective in treating panic as well as depression are the monoamine oxidase (MAO) inhibitors. Two of these drugs that the *Harvard Mental Health Letter* considers effective for panic include tranylcypromine (Parnate) and isocarboxazid (Marplan) ("What Are the Current," 2000, p. 2).

Sapolsky (1994) illustrates that these MAO inhibitors work in the same way as GABA works on serotonin. The MAO inhibitors block the reuptake of norepinephrine. Nonetheless, a dangerous side effect can occur. Norepinephrine is connected to the functioning of the sympathetic nervous system, which stimulates the body. One of the outcomes of this stimulation is the constriction of blood vessels, which in turn increases blood pressure (pp. 205-206). Consequently, the use of MAO inhibitors can be dangerous for someone with cardiovascular problems.

Psychological Approaches to Treating Panic Disorders

Behavioral Therapy, Cognitive-Behavioral Therapy, and Exposure Therapy

The American Psychological Association (2000) stated the following in an online public-affairs bulletin: "Most specialists agree that a combination of cognitive and behavioral therapies are the best treatment for panic disorder" (p. 4). Other sources indicating that a cognitive-behavioral approach is efficacious include Medscape (2000),

"Mental Health: Facts" (1999), Agras (1985), and Klerman et al. (1993).

Brown and Lempa (2000) stated that the two most effective forms of psychotherapy for anxiety disorders are *behavioral therapy* and *cognitive behavioral therapy*. First, the authors identified *behavioral therapy* as an approach which, "tries to change actions through techniques such as diaphragmatic breathing whereby slow, deep breaths are taken to reduce anxiety." Second, cognitive behavioral therapy is described as an approach to modify the thoughts of the patient. This therapy attempts to help the patient understand thinking patterns that trigger anxiety and, subsequently, redirect the reactions to the circumstances that cause anxiety. Finally, a collateral technique to the above approaches is *exposure therapy* through which, "people are very slowly exposed to the fearful situation until they become desensitized to it" (p. 6).

Brown and Lempa (2000) also cite the work of Dr. David Barlow (1990) at the State University of New York where he designed a treatment called panic control treatment. Components of this treatment include (1) redirected thinking, (2) the distinction and separation of somatic reactions such as hyperventilation and a rapid heartbeat from the stressor that creates panic, and (3) interoceptive exposure (p. 7).

Barlow (1992) commented on the interoceptive exposure model he created for the treatment of panic. He emphasized that the treatment "focuses on the panic attacks themselves rather than on agoraphobic avoidance" (pp. 3-4). One approach Barlow uses is to introduce feared somatic reactions such as hyperventilation and a rapid heartbeat in a structured setting. The patient experiences these somatic sensations through exercise and voluntary hyperventilation. When the feared somatic symptoms or combinations thereof are identified in this clinical setting, they become the focalization of treatment. Included with this treatment are exercises that produce derealization and depersonalization of the feared events.

It should be noted again that in the same article, Barlow advocates an approach to treating panic disorders which includes drug therapy along with the panic control techniques just described. Barlow believes it is a mistake to approach treatment from a "linear causal model." He sees psychology and biology inextricably tied together. Hence, Barlow considers the best approach for treating panic disorders to be a multidetermined causal model (p. 2).

A coda to this discussion on the cognitive-behavioral approach concerns some findings reported by Medscape (2000). According to this report, cognitive-behavioral therapy, which includes interoceptive exposure and cognitive restructuring, elicited a higher and longer-lasting rate of recovery than other forms of intervention as per Craske, Brown, and Barlow (1991, p. 3). Notwithstanding these results, Shear et al. (1994) found that comparative results between "manualized nonprescriptive treatment (NPT)" and cognitive-behavioral therapy (CBT) showed no significant differences (p. 6). Despite the equivalent results, however, the group that received CBT continued to show further improvement beyond a six-month monitoring period, while the group receiving manualized NPT showed a slight decline (pp. 6-7).

CONCLUSION

So there you have it: an overview of what has been researched and written in the realm of panic attacks, anxiety, phobias, the connection to depression and stress, and how all of this related to my personal experience with a panic meltdown. The overview is not exhaustive and, as is evident from the research, many loose ends to these phenomena have not been tied together. The quest for answers continues.

Within this matrix, Emil Authelet and I will explore the causes of panic in a different way. Drawing upon psychodynamic connections to my family of origin as well as the cognitive-behavioral principle of restructured thinking, we will add to the formula a spiritual dimension: panic can be the outcome of a person's inability to really believe and accept the unconditional love of God.

The time is now; the setting is the dawn of the twenty-first century; the story is of an adult caregiver who has a meltdown because of reactions to accumulated life stressors; the underlying cause is that within the adult is a frightened child who cannot subconsciously believe he is worthy of unconditional love—hence the recovery from panic begins with the resolution of childhood conflict and the restructuring of thinking to include the possibility that this adult has a right to be loved and accepted by other human beings, and that he has the right to be loved and accepted by God. The frightened child need not panic nor run any longer. This is the paradigm for this individual's story of recovery.

Before we embark on this exploration, Dr. David Betat will share his understanding of panic from the perspective of a physician with a deep faith in God.

Chapter 3

Clinical and Spiritual Perspectives on Anxiety, Panic Attacks, and the Malfunctioning of Our Brains: An Interview with Dr. David Betat

Daniel Langford

INTRODUCTION

David Betat was one of the two rescuers who helped pull me out of the "slough of despondency" and panic during the summer of 1999. Later, he agreed to be interviewed by me. When I reflected on this interview, I saw it as an illustration of a man who has fully integrated his Christian faith with his medical practice without apology. For those people who are not Christians, some of the material in this chapter may be difficult to embrace. Furthermore, Emil and I wrote this book from a Christian worldview. Our Christian heritage, despite the loose ends and tensions it creates in a world that worships pure science, makes us who we really are. Therefore, to deny our benchmark of faith is to deny the philosophical foundations upon which this book is written. It is my hope that those who read this chapter and the rest of the story can look beyond any reaction to our Christian worldview and find in the heart of the writing something to make life more understandable, fulfilling, and serene.

I would like to suggest reframing our story if Christianity is not your worldview. Not long ago, I was called into my boss's office at the middle school where I teach. The principal was very concerned because I had recited the Serenity Prayer and used the name of God during an in-house televised school program on conflict resolution and anger management. She reminded me that we were in a public school setting and that some people get very upset when the name of God is even mentioned. So I figured out how to alleviate the problem. During the next teaching session, I said, "May the Force be with you."

May the Force be with you when you read our story, and please apply what you will to your own model of spirituality.

In considering Dr. Betat's integration of his faith and medical practice, I was impressed with the simplicity through which he related his faith to medicine. William Hendricks (1980) would describe such an approach as a Hebrew model of the reading and interpretation of scripture, which is a "hear, see and obey" model (p. 65).

In contrast, I think of my own allegorical counterpart to the study of the Bible as we experienced it in seminary. The Bible became a cadaver on which we as seminary students performed an autopsy in a manner similar to that of a medical student who explores the innards of a dead human to find out how to best practice medicine on the living. We, as seminarians, took the Bible apart, dissected it into criticisms, settings in the life, biographies of the writers, nuances of language translations, obscurities of texts, and problems of applications to modern times.

In contrast, Dr. Betat did not perform such a theological autopsy when he spoke of his faith and quoted the scriptures. He quoted the biblical messages in their extant simplicity and made direct applications to his understanding and practice of medicine. I experienced some tension about this, maybe because I knew too much about the background of some of the passages that he used as references. Nevertheless, as I talked with Dr. Betat and heard him speak the Word, I realized that his very straightforward approach to the scriptures communicated truth that even science and human experience back up today.

Here is an example. Whether or not you believe that Noah really existed or that men and women lived to be 900 years old, like Methuselah, as recorded in the book of Genesis, you cannot get away from the scientific evidence that supports one of the passages related to the story of Noah and the Ark. According to Genesis 6:3, God said to Noah, "My spirit shall not abide in man forever, for he is flesh, but his days shall be a hundred and twenty years" (RSV). Isn't this true today? Few live to be 100 and only rarely do some men and women reach the age of 120.

So, when I interviewed Dr. Betat, I put away my Bible as a cadaver model. I sewed up the Bible, at least for the moment. I stuffed criticism, history, translation, and interpretation back into its body and took it off the autopsy table. What I did, instead, was listen to a man share his living faith with the life-giving words of scripture, the foundation of that faith. I listened for the ring of truth and how the understanding of God, the world, and medicine were expressed in the life and practice of one doctor who rescued me from intense psychological and emotional suffering. I hope you can do the same. Here is our dialogue.

A DIALOGUE WITH DAVID BETAT, MD

Primal Causes of the Fight-or-Flight Response and Contemporary Triggers of Panic Attacks

DANIEL LANGFORD: What I thought we would do is bounce around some of the things we talked about when I came in to see you during the time I was experiencing the panic attacks. I remember you stated last year that we as the human species are not improving biologically. In fact, you said you believe the human species is deteriorating both mentally and physically.

DR. DAVID BETAT: Our mental and physical capacities are not what they were two thousand years ago, if we were given the same set of circumstances and lived in those times.

DL: Is this because there is an overall deterioration in our genetic makeup as a human species?

DB: There has just been more time for genetic errors to become manifested. Because of this, the human organism taken as a whole over time is not working as well as it used to.

DL: You mentioned that panic attacks are an expression of a fight-or-flight response in the absence of a tangible threat or stressor. When we look at human life two thousand or three thousand years ago, when life was somewhat simpler, man in those times had only to be concerned about getting or growing food and protecting himself from wild animals or other human raiders. When I consider this relative simplicity, I am reminded of Robert Sapolsky's arguments [1994] for why zebras don't get ulcers. He said zebras are dealing with actual physical dangers and, consequently, can do something about those dangers immediately, such as running from a lion. He also talked about the humans of long ago who experienced chronic physical stressors, such as crop failures from locust attacks which resulted in six months of wandering to get enough food to survive. Despite these pressures, Sapolsky argues that in such sustained disasters, non-Westernized humans and most other mammals handle the bodily responses to these real stressors very well [p. 5]. Fight-or-flight responses kick in and the mammal or ancient human could actually do something about the problems.

DB: It is true. We face problems in modern society from which we can neither run nor fight.

DL: I believe some fight-or-flight responses we have to modern stressors have nothing to do with real danger, such as an attacking lion or crops ruined by a plague of locusts.

DB: Well, it's a different kind of danger. The danger may not be a lion in our modern society, but there is a danger of some sort as we perceive things in our minds. When a lion chases you, you have a clear understanding of what is threatening you, but with something like a panic attack, there are more subtle things affecting you rather than something obvious like a lion. For example, panic attacks can result from an accumulation of stress and thinking ahead. When a lion attacks you, you are thinking about what you need to do right at that particular moment. However, a panic attack can be related to future fears. We might worry about whether we will have enough money to pay the utility bills next month. We might worry whether or not we will be alive next year because of this or that. These future worries could trigger anxiety and panic. We try to accumulate all the futures on our back in the present, and that can trigger something. But these are not the only triggers for panic attacks.

Environment, Heredity, and Brain Chemistry As Triggers of Panic

DL: Concurrently, you mentioned that heredity can contribute to panic attacks. During your assessment last year, when I came to you for help, you asked about my family history.

DB: We don't know for sure how much genetics and how much environment contribute to the problems of anxiety and panic attacks, but we do know for sure that both of these factors together contribute to the problems. They are not separate from each other. There is very little in life that is purely environmental or purely genetic. Some things are primarily one or the other. However, environment and genetics almost always influence each other regardless of the degree.

DL: What you are saying reminds me of the training I had to become a social worker. We were taught to look for multiple factors that affect a human being and his or her current circumstances. We were taught to look at the biopsychosocial components of a person's situation—and I am thinking we could also include the spiritual component. All of these dynamics work together. Related to all of this, I would like to ask you some questions about the influences of environment and heredity as they relate to my experiences with panic and anxiety.

When I came to you as a patient in August 1999, no doubt you remember I could hardly sit in the examination room because of the darkness and the closed door. Nonetheless, about two months after those initial visits with you, things began to settle down around me. My environment became less stressful. My panic reactions began to lessen significantly, which I attribute to improved life circumstances and the benefits of medication. Concurrently, I decided to discontinue the use of antianxiety medication, as I felt I no longer needed it.

Nonetheless, even though the distressful panic attacks I experienced a year ago are gone, there are still things that bother me even today. For example, I can't stand being crammed in a tight space on an airplane. It is not fear of flying that persists; it is the fear of being trapped in an enclosed space. I am not afraid to fly—just give me an aisle seat so that a food tray is not blocking my ability to get out and move around.

So, here is what I am asking you: I am no longer experiencing the terror of panic that occurred in the summer of 1999. Yet there appear to be residual symptoms that persist. The discomfort of a window seat on a plane is one example. Also, I experienced a brief déjà vu of the panic I experienced in 1999. During the middle of July 2000, I woke out of a deep sleep at about 2:00 a.m., and I thought for sure I was going into a panic meltdown again. How-ever, the experience was transitory, and I have not had problems since. What do you think about this? Was this an organic or biolog-ical reaction, since there were no apparent stressors?

DB: It may well have been a biological reaction. However, if you go to your spouse, you might discover that there were stressors you did not even know about.

DL: Since you mentioned that, I do remember that I was waging war at the time with gophers in my vegetable garden. My wife stated that she saw I was using up too much emotional energy over a problem that was not that big of a deal. She reminded me that the garden was not an extension of my personhood. I did take her ad-vice, "chilled out," and also found a way to get rid of the gophers. This is sort of like the locust plague we discussed previously.

Next, regarding the discomfort I just described for cramped spaces such as airplane seats, do you think our brains become "hardwired" to react to certain triggers that generate anxiety or panic?

DB: Certain things do trigger a panic attack for some people. For ex-ample, enclosed spaces will trigger a panic attack for some people. I have also seen something else. Some persons can go spelunking [cave exploring] when they are teenagers, but when these same persons are older, they develop claustrophobia and can no longer do this activity.

DL: Why is that?

DB: We don't know. We don't have a complete explanation for that.

DL: Does brain chemistry change with age?

DB: I think it could be a combination of both the environment and brain chemistry. For instance, if you had a bad experience with spelunking and got stuck in a crevice, and it took all day for some-one to rescue you, you could develop a fear of cramped spaces and never go spelunking again.

The Bible and the Deterioration of the Human Species

DL: I would like to change directions a little and reconsider your bib-lical perspectives on what you see as a universal deterioration of human beings over time as well as the general decline in the ability of our species to cope with the pressures and contaminants of our contemporary world. Specifically, how does your faith integrate with your medical knowledge in explaining such a malady as panic attacks?

DB: I don't know if the concept of panic attacks ever occurs in the ancient Hebrew and Greek writings. Nevertheless, there were obviously people who were stressed in biblical times too. I also think that in those cultures and in those times that psychiatric diagnoses were considered to be very negative, almost as bad as leprosy. This is true in some cultures today. You don't get a diagnosis of a psychiatric disorder, because you might not be able to get anyone to marry you or marry your children. Essentially, there is still plenty of stigmata connected to a psychiatric diagnosis. So, I think such things as panic attacks are not mentioned in the Bible outright. This is not to say that people in biblical times did not have panic attacks. Nonetheless, because such things were so stigmatized, they were probably not written about.

The Effects of Sin

DB: So, we must consider God, who says he is willing to heal people, but most important, God wants to heal people of their sinful natures, their sinfulness. This gets into the whole process of sanctification and justification. Parallel to healing from sin, God also heals people of their physical maladies, too. That was Christ's point of suffering on the cross: Christ died for human physical maladies as well as for human behavior.

When considering all of this, I think that someone who has a depressive, social anxiety, or panic disorder with hereditary triggers out of his or her control is like the blind man in the New Testament. Jesus' disciples asked, "Who sinned? His parents or him?" [John 9:2]. So it is the same here. No one has sinned just because you have a panic disorder or a depression disorder. That does not mean that you are a bad person. You did not necessarily do something bad in your life that caused this. At this point we go back to genetics. I was born blind because there was a chromosome that did not work very well during the process of embryonic genesis. The same thing goes for our brains, which are just as susceptible to defects as the rest of our bodies. Some people are just born with defects.

DL: This would be a good time to go back of the idea of the Fall or the introduction of sin as we read in the book of Genesis in the Old Testament.

DB: God says clearly in the book of Exodus that unto the third and fourth generation will I visit the sins of the parents [Exodus 20:5]. That passage really implies that genetics are quite significant in the happenstance of physical and mental problems in the lives of people. For example, we can see that if a parent is an alcoholic, the children have the potential of becoming alcoholics themselves. Even if the first generation of these alcoholic parents become tee-totalers, the generation that follows can become alcoholics because of the genetic weakness that is carried on. So then the grand-children become alcoholics.

DL: Hence, a genetic problem might skip one generation and show up in another.

DB: Yes. You as a person might say, because of environmental forces, "I am not going to drink." You make this decision because you see what your parents went through. However, the grandchildren may not have experienced this firsthand, but they still have the genes in them. Thus, if these grandchildren get a hold of a little alcohol, they may become rapidly hooked—more so than someone who does not come from a family with an alcoholic background.

DL: Would you describe all of this as genetic deterioration? Furthermore, is this your position based upon a spiritual decline of humans or upon scientific principles of thermodynamics that contend that all matter decays over time?

DB: I base my position upon a spiritual decline. I think by the grace of God we all can attain a higher spiritual level in any generation. We cannot do this alone; we need the grace of God. Nevertheless, I do not think that any generation has bridged the gap between God and man since the Fall.

DL: The book of Genesis has the story of mankind's fall, and the focus of the story is Adam and Eve's choice to eat fruit from a tree that gives them knowledge of good and evil. This story does not fit neatly into the thinking of our scientific age, and I don't understand all the mystery and loose ends that swirl around the account. Nevertheless, if I understand Genesis 3 correctly, because Adam and Eve chose to eat of the tree that gave them God's knowledge of good and evil, death was introduced into the human experience. According to this passage, if the tree's fruit had not been eaten, we would not experience death as we do now. But human beings do experience death, and the decay that comes with aging so far appears to be inevitable.

DB: As I said before, we as humans are more prone to problems as a species because of deterioration over time. This really makes sense from a creationist standpoint that we are going downhill and not uphill—unless Christ intervenes. The Bible expresses the concept of the world as a diamond that is wearing down; a garment that is wearing out. The earth is like a wine sack that has gotten older. [See Isaiah 24 and Isaiah 51:6.] This whole planet is wearing out. We can't sustain six billion people on the earth. If we keep growing with the population, we will run out of potable water, places to grow food, and even places to put our houses.

DL: I read a recent news article about a desert area in China that had lost all the water in a water table. Wells were dry, and the people there can no longer farm, much less survive.

DB: We have seen it here in the United States. If you pump enough water, you will pump a huge aquifer down and increase salinity. Related to all of this discussion, there are some who study the Old Testament who believe that there may have been several billion people living at the time of Noah and the flood. This would make sense if you do the mathematics. People in the time of Noah lived to be nine hundred years old. So if you had a child every nine months, you could have a lot of kids.

DL: Do you believe that nine-hundred-year life spans, which were documented in the book of Genesis, reflect the actual years people lived in those times?

DB: God says in Genesis that He repented of making mankind with long life spans. What was happening was really sad. So God decided to limit man's life span to one hundred twenty years [Genesis 6:1-5]. The best any human being can do since the flood is live to one hundred twenty years. Every once in a while, we see someone who lives to be one hundred and five, and rarely do we see anyone living to one hundred and twenty years. The human genes have been so polluted since the flood that it is going to be tough for any person to reach such life spans as one hundred and twenty years.

DL: I have heard and read of a few people in other parts of the world that have reached ages of one hundred and nineteen. I don't know if there has been a person to live as long in the United States.

DB: I think we are seeing the effects of sin. God has been merciful by allowing us to have mechanical tools, such as tractors, to assist us with the growing of food. If we did not have technology, we would not be able to provide enough food for everyone. Even though we hate to admit we have to use such stuff, pesticides, herbicides, and fertilizers have enabled us to grow the food we need to feed the world.

DL: I would like to explore the concept of sin with you and the effects of sin. One translation of sin from both Hebrew and Greek origins is "missing the mark." There is another idea for sin as being negative behavior or acts of a person. When you think of the concept of sin, what are you thinking of?

DB: Are you asking if a panic attack is a sin?

DL: That is not my question. We have discussed the world as wearing out like a diamond. If we say that the deterioration of the world is caused by sin, what are you referring to? Are you referring to the destructive behavior of human beings directly, or are you referring to the repercussions of human evil which has precipitated such things as genetic breakdown and the degeneration of human life?

DB: Sin is a composite of both the negative actions of human beings and the repercussions that follow. Sin is a self-destructive process. Eventually, if God does not intervene, sin, like a fire, will burn itself out. It will consume everything in its path, including human beings [Romans 6:23]. God has to demonstrate to the universe that if you follow the devil's plan and you follow the way of sin, sin basically destroys itself.

DL: Are we looking at sin just at the Fall in the Garden of Eden, or do we look at sin as an ongoing process where man continues to make choices that result in negative outcomes that affect not only himself but the community he lives in?

DB: I believe we as humans choose a course of action that affects us now and will eventually affect us in the future.

The End of the World

DL: What does your personal faith teach you about the downward tailspin or deterioration the world is experiencing? What will happen at the very end?

DB: The Bible says that time will be cut short. I believe that God will intervene before the entire world is destroyed. If you believe the book of Revelation, there will be trumpets blowing and much havoc toward the end before Christ comes, but Christ will intervene before the entire world goes up in smoke.

DL: What happens to us?

DB: Do you mean what happens to Christians?

DL: Yes.

DB: That's becoming somewhat theological. Are you asking what will happen at the very end?

DL: Yes.

DB: A lot of people speculate how physical that will be [the new age of Christ's rule], but the book of Revelation is real specific and mentions four living creatures [Revelation 4:6-10]—so you would think there would be some physicalness to it. That age may be a different physical reality than what we know now. We may have a slightly different nervous system, and we won't be experiencing physical pain. For sure, we won't be experiencing any mental or emotional pain.

Nonetheless, there will be solemnity during the judgment time. This is where Seventh Day Adventists may depart from the beliefs of other Christians. We feel there is a thousand-year period where the saints will be in heaven [Daniel 7; Revelation 20], and they, along with Christ, will be opening up the books of the people who are not in heaven. This will be a solemn or sad time because there will be many who have not accepted the blood of Christ who will not have a place, and you will recognize that certain members of your own family and friends will not make it. This will be a sad note, but this is a necessary job, and people have to be convinced that God is fair.

DL: Thus, in your tradition of faith, do you believe in a literal, physical return of Jesus Christ to judge the world?

DB: Yes, and along with this return of Christ, I believe we will be given new bodies that will be incorruptible.

The Practice of Medicine and Biblical Faith

DL: I would like to ask you a question related to your beliefs that you just shared with me. Suppose you went to a convention with other physicians who are your peers. Further, you expressed these ideas with some physicians who had no faith. Consider that you were attempting to communicate your faith to doctors who had no Christian beliefs and merely saw the human body as a natural machine that could be treated with pills, surgery, or whatever. Such physicians see life only from a naturalistic, nonfaith perspective. I think you understand that if you share the things we shared with someone who neither believes in God nor accepts the traditions of Christian faith, this stuff sounds really bizarre to such a person, and many would find it hard to understand how a person who is knowledgeable of medicine, such as yourself, could also have these seemingly incongruous religious convictions. So, how do you synchronize a scientific/medical understanding of human beings with the tenets of your faith? How do you put these together?

DB: I cannot speculate upon how my colleagues who do not believe as I do might react to my faith. Nevertheless, you may realize that we have limitations as physicians. We cannot solve every problem, whether it be mental, emotional, physical, or spiritual. Therefore, we who are believing doctors must rely on a higher power to assist us with the care of our patients.

I do not know how atheistic physicians handle the dilemmas they face. Some philosophers say that the power is within you. You just have to get it out. Nevertheless, from my perspective as a Christian, you have to go to God, to that higher power, to have the ultimate healing. You might be able to give a pill to battle bacteria in the bloodstream, and you might be able to give a pill that helps shift the neurochemicals in the brain so that a person has less pain, anxiety, or depression. But, ultimately, it is still God who does the final healing.

DL: So when you work with your patients, you practice with the perspective that you are not working alone; you work with God.

DB: Furthermore, I believe that whether or not an individual acknowledges God in the healing event does not change the fact in my mind that God is still the healer.

Do you remember the story of Jesus healing the ten lepers [Luke 17:11-19]? How many of those ten turned back and praised God?

DL: Just one.

DB: Only one out of ten acknowledged the healing, even though all experienced the healing. Despite the advances provided by our modern treatments, there are still few that acknowledge God is the source of these medical advances.

Seventh Day Adventists and the Medical Mission

DL: The next question I want to ask you is meant to satisfy my curiosity about your Seventh Day Adventist faith. I have met a number of Seventh Day Adventists in my career as a Baptist minister, and I have studied a little of your church's history. Nevertheless, I have always been intrigued that Seventh Day Adventists play such a significant role in modern-day medicine. Why is medicine so important to Seventh Day Adventists?

DB: The center of our involvement in medicine is that Christ spent a greater part of his ministry as a healer. Hence, if you don't take care of the physical needs of humanity, people will not be open to their spiritual needs.

If your stomach is empty and you have sores on your body, it is very hard to listen to a preacher, because you are uncomfortable physically. Therefore, as I just said, if you treat a person's physical needs, such a person will be much more open to spiritual needs.

It makes sense to me that God wants to heal all of our infirmities—spiritual and physical. We will not live in these decrepit bodies for the next ten million years. God has delivered us from that. Nevertheless, God's primary goal is to deliver us spiritually.

DL: Let me return again to the issue that aroused my curiosity regarding Seventh Day Adventists and medicine. The Catholics are the only other Christian group that appears to be immersed in medicine and the care of the sick to the degree that you as Seventh Day Adventists embrace medicine as a vocation. This is not to say that other denominations are not caring for the sick. Many denominations have hospitals and medical centers as a part of their focus of ministry. So, I am not minimizing the contributions of other churches to medicine and the healing arts. Nevertheless, medicine appears to me to be one of the most important missions of the Seventh Day Adventists. I want to know why.

DB: We have the great commission in Matthew 28:18-20. The great commission is to go out and baptize everyone from every nation. Medicine is our way as a church to reach other cultures. Some cultures will not accept a preacher in the same way that they will accept a hospital or physician.

DL: Where does medical emphasis come in to the history of the Adventist churches? Is it an early or late component of your faith?

DB: I would consider medicine to be the focal point of the modern Adventist movement. Medicine has had a significant role in the launching of the church's ministry since its very inception. Health is a very effective way to reach people in groups.

DL: So why do you want to reach all the people you do through your medical practice?

DB: If you want me to be blunt about it, our primary purpose is to proselytize our faith. But why do I want to do that? I want every human being possible to be in heaven with me. The ultimate goal for me is that every human being I come in contact with would ultimately join me in the kingdom of God. My ultimate goal is that my patients will respond to Christ.

The Pressure of Being a Doctor

DL: As we conclude our discussion, I wonder about something else that you experience every day as a doctor. You are immersed daily in the sufferings of human beings. How do you cope with this pressure, and how do you resolve the disappointments of not being able to see everyone get the healing they need or want? Fit this into your earlier observation that we are in a world that is sliding downhill and the human condition is not getting better. Are you standing in the gap—are you like the young boy holding back the ocean with his finger in the dike?

DB: My hope is to get some people out of the path of the slide altogether. I realize I can't help everyone or change the course of the world. I hope to help a few.

A Healer

DL: Setting aside the end of time and all those things that come with this end, you did something for me in the present that was very important. For at least a moment in time, you helped me alleviate some distressing feelings of anxiety and panic through your compassion and medical knowledge. My quality of life has been improved. Undoubtedly, you do the same for many others—even those who may reject your invitation to a spiritual reconciliation with God.

DB: I believe God cares for all people, believers or not, and wants humans to experience life with a minimum of pain and suffering. The Third Letter of John [verse 2] in the New Testament has these lines: "I pray that all may go well with you and that you may be in health" [RSV]. God wants us to be in good physical health as well as good spiritual health. God promised this to the Israelites in the Old Testament: "If you will diligently hearken to the voice of the Lord your God, and do that which is right in his eyes, and give heed to his commandments and keep all his statutes, I will put none of the diseases upon you which I put upon the Egyptians; for I am the Lord, your healer" [Exodus 15:26]. There are the words and ministry of Jesus back in the Old Testament, too.

DL: We are all going to die, but, again, healing whatever afflictions we have provides relief and an enhanced enjoyment of life, if only for a moment in time. I do not have the words to describe how grateful I was when I saw you last year and experienced the relief from the panic attacks I was going through. It would have been hell for me not to find relief, and I could not bear the prospect of going through weeks and months of this emotional and psychic pain without some release. Yes, I am going to die, but it is important for the thousand moments in time that precede my death that life be, as much as possible, pain free and enjoyable.

DB: I think that is important, and also your perception and experience of good health may determine when you die as well.

DL: I believe Kathryn Kuhlman once said that the experiences of healing we receive from God in this lifetime give us a glimpse of what heaven will be like. Kathryn Kuhlman recognized that spiritual rebirth—reconciliation—was the most important event in a person's life. Nevertheless, for most of us, the experience of physical healing is our most urgent need. Thus, the healing touch from God gets our attention and gives us a glimpse of heaven.

DB: Sometimes it is hard for us to perceive God, because he is not an entity that we can perceive with our five senses. Therefore, if we have a physical healing through the ministrations of a healing professional and/or through prayer, we are given the hope that there are better things to come. We can also experience this in a spiritual realm that cannot always be put down in words. Our spiritual experiences as well can also be a piece of heaven. I think our spiritual experiences are more important than our physical experiences.

There are plenty of things we cannot explain. How was Stephen able to sing when he was stoned to death [Acts 7]? I think that he was so connected with God that he did not experience the pain of those stones being hurled at him. I think such experiences are possible even for people today.

DL: Acts 7:56 states that Stephen said, "I see the heavens opened, and the Son of man standing at the right hand of God" [RSV].

DB: That was the way he left this life, and it was evident that God was with him.

DL: Let's take a moment to look upon a theme in the philosophy of existentialism. I explored the ideas of existentialism briefly in my training to become a social worker as well as the teaching I received in seminary. One of the themes in existential thought is that we as humans live between two events in life that are out of our control. The beginning event is birth, and the inevitable, ending event is death.

DB: I think we can control somewhat when we die by how we care for our bodies.

DL: I understand. But death as a final event in human life will come to all of us, and that inevitability is out of our control. Nevertheless, existentialism looks at life between the curtains of birth and death and asks how can life be the fullest, most enjoyable, and most meaningful for every human being. Maslow's concept of self-actualization—to be as fully human and fully alive as a giving person to self and the world—is an example of this theme. What are your thoughts about this?

DB: My belief in Christ is what allows me to reach such a potential. I do not think I can reach such completeness apart from my relationship to Christ. I think all of us have missed some opportunities along the way to develop our lives more fully. If we were perfect, then we would not miss any opportunities. Nevertheless, God uses imperfect vessels to move his work forward.

DL: Consequently, do you see yourself as a doctor in the classic New Testament translation of *aggelos* [angel], as a messenger of good news and ambassador of Jesus Christ?

DB: Yes, but at the same time, I see myself as an imperfect conduit. Sometimes the message gets there through me, but it is frequently imperfect because we as doctors do not have all the answers for everyone's problems.

DL: Thank you again, Dr. Betat, for all you did for me.

Chapter 4

The Frightened Child Hiding
Behind the Facade of an Adult

Emil Authelet

THE DAN LANGFORD I FIRST MET

My first impression of Dan when I met him some nine years ago was of a laid-back, conscientious, sensitive human being who loved working with people. I thought he would make a great pastor if he were allowed to meet people where they are and help them reach where they need to be. I could picture him taking his people along with him on a journey into spiritual and emotional maturity, addressing their needs as they went. If the new church start we American Baptists were planning for Crescent City, California, was to be a success, he would be an excellent candidate for the role of pastor. We knew Crescent City would present many problems, because the anticipated new arrivals would center around an expanding community hosting one of the state's largest new prisons. The prison would house long-term, hard-core offenders, and the community would absorb their families. We needed a pastor who could fit among these families, one with a good balance between spiritual and psychological growth.

This impression was also shared by Robert Rasmussen, the Executive Minister for the American Baptist Churches of the West. Bob knew Dan from Dan's earlier years as a pastor at Gualala, California. Bob vacationed in that area every summer; on those occasions, Dan was his pastor.

Not only was Dan selected to lead that new church in Crescent City, but in the process he and I became colleagues as well as friends. We hit it off right from the start, and our friendship soon grew beyond the work to sharing in three major areas: our concerns over ministry and needy persons, our family needs and concerns for our kids, and our shared thoughts about the whole field of relational theology— combining the best of biblical insights with the development of a biblical and psychological worldview of relationships. Since we were often many miles apart geographically, many of our conversations were by phone and written correspondence, but they were regular and often long. Praying for each other was also part of our relationship.

As caregivers, we shared much in common and often extended this caregiving to each other, depending on whose need arose first. I valued these times together, for we both spoke from a common experience and shared need. The actual face-to-face times were extended as much as possible so that we could share ideas and thoughts from our mutual readings and research into relational theology.[1]

STRUGGLES WITH A MISSION

The work at Crescent City took several twists and turns that neither of us anticipated, but I always knew Dan's decisions were well thought out, prayed over, and in the best interests of the people involved. Nevertheless, the anticipated influx of new residents to Crescent City did not happen, and those attracted to the new church brought more problems than any one fellowship could handle. Dan soon found that like begets like, and the people the work attracted were not stable enough to build on, so the load really fell on his shoulders and heart. It was obvious the work would never become self-supporting, and Dan had to carry the financial load as well when other funding was exhausted or withdrawn. He was doing the work and paying the bills at the same time. The three sponsoring churches did not see the potential of a crystal cathedral in the floundering mission, so each began to abandon ship. The sponsors' criticisms of Dan's methods were like telling a drowning sailor to take a deep breath and all would be well. They understood nothing of the people attending or of the deep needs represented; they just wanted him to replicate their fellowships, even though Dan did not have the supportive congregational base the sponsoring churches had. Through all of this, I saw both compassion and frustration in Dan: compassion for the people being served and frustration for those who did not even care to try to understand.

Crisis in the Workplace and a Necessary Move

Dan's so-called secular employment at a nursing home was an extension of his heart for ministry wherever and to whomever. To him, the church and the everyday world of work were both contexts and places for ministry: he ministered in both settings. Both he and his wife Diana did what they did out of a single heart, and this landed them right in the middle of controversy, because others preferred darkness to light and profits to caring. Because of the negative circumstances that developed at the nursing home, it became obvious that Dan and Diana needed to leave the area, which also meant leaving the work at American Baptist Fellowship. I supported their decision; it was the right thing for them to do. God's vineyard is vast and varied. He would use them elsewhere.

Throughout the long search and the transition from Crescent City to Lakeport, Dan did what needed to be done and did it well. His faith was pruned and strengthened; his spirit remained positive and bright. Throughout all this turmoil, he was completing his book, *The Pastor's Family*, and keeping his family focus intact. Dan and Diana together were doing what needed to be done. Their personal disappointments in leaving their new home were taken in stride as part of the greater adventure of following God's leading.

WAR IN THE CLASSROOM

Lakeport, California, brought new challenges as well as some familiar ones. Dan's return to the classroom was a natural for him, but he was totally unprepared for what he encountered. All the old expectations of kids wanting to learn and do something about their futures were absent. This was a war zone. The students were not getting what they wanted from the staff and administration, and they were making their unhappiness felt. Dan was their target for making their needs, frustrations, and disappointments known. Hardest of all was the reality that a man of deep compassion for youth and their real needs was being kept at bay and never allowed to reach out except to a very few. The students were not about to give Dan a chance to get close to them. The administration told him to "hang in and keep trying," but that message never got through to the kids themselves.

A Decision to Leave and a Choice to Stay

During this crisis, calls between Dan and me were frequent and the prayers were urgent. In the spring of 1999, things came to a head, and Dan was ready to walk away from it all. He was being as realistic as he could: his teaching was not working; he was being pulled under; and he saw no real possibility of changing the students. I am not sure how he was able to hang in as long as he did. When he finally found the inner freedom to leave, walk away from it, and seek work elsewhere, at the same time, he also found the inner strength and freedom to remain in that classroom until the end of the school year.

THE CRISIS OF THE INNER CHILD

With the end of the school year, there came a relaxation of tension—physically, mentally, psychologically, and spiritually. He had made it through. But summer passes, and before you know it fall arrives. August brought this realization to Dan's Inner Child's full attention. The Inner Child of the Past had been pulled through a wringer he did not want to experience ever again, and now he was about to reenter that crucible. The Inner Child pushed the panic button and brought Dan's whole world to a halt: "You're not going to drag me back into that crucible and put me through that again!"

Being unable to verbalize this for fear of the outcome, such as being branded a failure, the Inner Child resorted to the only means he had to get Dan's attention. He pushed the button marked "Adrenaline Rush—Anxiety Overload!" and stood back to see what would happen. What did happen came from the top of Dan's head to the bottom of his feet: anxiety and panic took over. Every alarm went off, as if foreign missiles were seen approaching and no shelter was in sight, so the alarm screamed, "Run! Run and run until you cannot run anymore. There has to be some means of escape!"

Familiar Chords of Crisis

Dan's call to me during this time of crisis was filled with panic seeking to express itself in very rational terms so he might grasp the reality of what was happening but at the same time fearing no answer could be found. He was trying hard to be in control, while his gut was telling him all was lost. It was as though he was striking a tuning fork in Lakeport and a chord in me began to vibrate in Vallejo. I knew exactly what was happening because I had been there during my collegiate days, and the vibrations were as clear as they had been years ago within myself. I could tell him I knew what he was feeling, for I had felt the same; it signified that Dan had lost control of his normal composure and little Dan had taken over with his inability to handle all that had been going on.

The Frightened Child Hiding Behind the Adult

The frightened little Child had been hiding behind Dan the Adult.[2] He was now trying to get Dan's attention with fear and anxiety and anger about the unfairness and pain of the situation. Worse yet, he was dwelling on self-blame for his failure, as he perceived it. The Inner Child is a master at self-blame.[3]

Payback to the Frightened Inner Child

Dan, with Diana's encouragement, was doing all the right things to help himself. First, he was checked out physically to see whether an imbalance might be causing the panic attacks and to know that all was well physically. Then he took a psychological/spiritual inventory and called me for my input. He also sought counsel from trusted friends and colleagues in the area. From these resources, he got what he needed to start regaining control as the Adult. He had a debt he owed to little Dan that he had to pay. He needed to help him, to understand what all this had cost him, to be there for him no matter what, and to let him know he did not have to go back into that crucible and endure all that pain again. The past year had robbed little Dan of all he cherished, and now it was time to give him something back. He also owed himself a change of thinking, for his negative thoughts were leading to negative feelings and negative actions. He was seeing himself as failing and, worse, as a failure. There was a lot of anger toward others who had failed him, and he was not able to place this blame where it belonged. The blame was getting swallowed up and dumped on little Dan.

Family-of-Origin Issues

Swallowed anger always leads to depression. These feelings were rooted in the family-of-origin issues Dan had been keeping the lid on for years. They started to surface during the writing of his book, *The Pastor's Family,* but not enough to be resolved. They were still there, suppressed and under control, until the adrenaline surge of panic forced them to surface with a vengeance. They needed to be dealt with, and only a transformation in thinking—from delusion and prejudice to reality—would do. To turn him in that direction, I first shared with Dan how I saw him as a person and how God sees him, then recommended he get a copy of John Powell's (1976) little book *Fully Human, Fully Alive.* I recommended that he begin reading it and that we discuss his discoveries in follow-up calls. Between the physical help and then the rational/emotive and spiritual help, Dan was on his way to change and recovery.

A NEW LEVEL OF SELF-AWARENESS

I knew Dan well enough to know that all you have to do is help him get pointed in the right direction and he will do the rest. What he needed most was to share all the compassion he has for others with himself. As Jesus said, "Love others as you love yourself" (Matthew 19:19; Mark 12:31; Luke 10:27). It was time for Dan to love himself in new and deeper ways. The caregiver had to learn how to care better for himself. He was not crazy, nor was he going crazy. But he was moving to a new level of self-awareness that would deepen his compassion for others experiencing anxiety and fear.

Here was a man who had recently earned the advanced degree of doctor of ministries, was a published author, had taught in a hornet's nest and survived, had worked with many people facing critical emotional and psychological needs, had a family in which he was loved and admired, and had professional colleagues who honored him as a person and as a professional, yet he still saw himself as a failure as he had as a kid growing up within a highly dysfunctional family. Having taken the responsibility for holding that family together, it was easy for him to fall back into that role and accept the responsibility for all that had and had not happened during the school year. He felt that receiving his doctorate was a fluke. He felt that if people really knew him, they would think differently about him, and that God was using him in some lives but only because no one else was there at that moment. This was all rooted in little Dan, the Inner Child, and his delusions had never been corrected. Now it was time for some reality testing.

As I hung up the phone after that initial call that August, my prayer for Dan was twofold. I prayed that God would be allowed to quiet his mind and heart so that he could begin to see what had happened and why, and seek the radical transformation of thought that would allow him to let go of the Inner Child's delusions and allow the Inner Adult to embrace reality. The other prayer was of thanksgiving that Dan and I had built a level of trust between us which allowed for honesty, compassion, and mutual affirmation to flow freely in and through the issues we shared. Just as I had resonated with his crisis, so he resonated with what I shared that had worked for me. Otherwise, I would have been in the car heading for Lakeport to be beside him until the real answer came.

RECOVERY

The crisis began to pass as Dan worked hard on his thinking patterns and how they had affected his self-perception. He had fallen into that pit devotional writers refer to as "the dark night of the soul." As he continued to focus on his family-of-origin work, it became more evident that areas of unfinished work had blindsided him when he needed it least. These issues needed to be faced, worked through, and put to rest where they belonged—in the past. Dan was working on an inner reconciliation between Dan the Adult and little Dan, the Inner Child of the Past. The negative emotions that surfaced for Dan were all indicators of what John Powell calls "malignant misconceptions" in how we perceive ourselves. We live out those perceptions. They become our sense of reality by which we judge all things. They must be tested against reality and updated when they fail the test. I love Dan because he is worth loving. He needed to see himself that way also and extend that love to his real self. It was time for the old to go and the new to dawn.

God Sees Us with Eyes of Love

None of us will ever know ourselves fully as God sees us, but we can gain enough clues to build a self-perception that aids us rather than sabotages us. Dan was sabotaging himself. His journey needed to take him to new insights that are based in the reality of his own true worth.

Self-Discovery and the Caregiver

All caregivers have participated in the journey of others, but not all have made a successful inner journey for themselves, within themselves. This inner journey is what makes caregivers what they most need to be—people who can truly resonate with the pain of another, knowing it is that person's pain they are feeling and not their own, and responding in empathy and compassion to that person's deep need. This is what caregiving is all about. God uses caregivers' personal journeys to forge the kinds of help He wants to offer all humankind.

Some lessons we learn from books and academic pursuits. Some come from life and from the ups and downs we experience as we go along. Some come from the wisdom and insights of others' journeys. But the unique lessons that become most meaningful to us are the ones circumstances may force us into. God meets us right in the middle and does His special work in our lives that could not have been learned in any other way. However, as in childbirth, the pain is worth the results. New life has been birthed within us—and through us to others. This book is about Dan's journey and the gift of caring he shares. Not only is it the fruit of his own journey, it is a journey shared because he was willing to do the hard work needed to make it through. Self-delusions do not let go easily.

Chapter 5

The Healing of the Frightened Child

Emil Authelet

INTRODUCTION

The unexpected happens. When it does, it has a way of getting our full attention. An accident, some kind of heartache, a breach of friendship, or a sudden panic attack can bring us to full attention and rivet us to the moment. It can be one of these moments that leave us forever altered. It can also be a time when God captures our full attention and we are left wondering how we could have been so blind-sighted. Such a God-moment gripped Dan as a result of a panic attack resulting from a floating anxiety that encompassed everything. What the attack did was bring him to full attention and God was waiting in the wings for this opportunity to speak. What He would say is exactly what Dan needed to hear.

Beneath the Surface of Our Consciousness

When things are working well, at least on the surface, we drift through our days often totally oblivious to what may be lurking just beneath the surface of our consciousness. These days can stretch into weeks, months, and years—even into decades. No stress, no pain, thus no real questions such as, "What might be waiting from an unfin-ished past that might interrupt, disrupt, or, worse yet, erupt?" The more years we live in this unexamined state, the more we tend to as-sume nothing is unresolved. We were affected long ago by a child-hood that may have been anything but enjoyable, but that was de-cades ago, and we may not even remember that past or want to. But it is there: all it takes is the right crisis, the right amount of inner pres-sure, and the volcano can blow. Some people learn to control the volcano so that instead of erupting, it simply oozes hot scorching lava in almost every relationship they encounter. This oozing lava appears as anger, fault finding, or feelings of rejection. People with these unresolved childhood issues tend to put the blame on others for their inability to form satisfying relationships.

Unresolved Issues of the Inner Child

Dan had issues to work through; some he had already conquered. What he failed to see were the unresolved issues regarding little Dan, the Inner Child of the Past. Dan struggled with a low level of self-worth and, at times, a low level of self-esteem. But being a "rescuer," he focused on others and rarely on himself. When he put his Inner Child through the crucible of the distressing school year with the "war zone" of his hostile classroom, he failed to see its toll on himself and especially on the Inner Child, who could not cope with such challenges. What a place for a rescuer to be in—surrounded by a group wanting anything but rescuing! The Child had been put on hold for a year while Dan the Adult struggled with survival needs. What about little Dan and his feelings of abandonment? Little Dan was being used and abused, just as he had been in the past, when he was a real child in a highly dysfunctional world—the only world he knew.

Panic Generated by the Inner Child

Little Dan felt anger and panic: "Here I am again! I didn't understand it the first time—I'm totally confused about what is going on this time—and I want out!" So little Dan got big Dan's full attention with a panic attack that was like tugging the ring in the nose of a bull; with it Dan the Adult was being led down a path that was extremely painful and scary, but he could not stop the journey. As fast as little Dan ran, he still could not outrun the panic.

The panic surfaced during August 1999 because no classroom, class, or administration had to be pleased, no "war zone" had to be survived, and August was a safe time. Little Dan gave that ring a twist, and Adult Dan came to full attention. "Now you will listen to me, or else!" said little Dan.

Not only was the past still there, it was in full control. Little Dan, with all his delusions and fears, was in total control of Adult Dan. In the night, when everything closes in, Dan was overwhelmed by the fear and pain and panic that little Dan brought to the surface and, consequently, Adult Dan's fight-or-flight mechanism went into high gear. Dan ran. All the negative thoughts and fears and unresolved conflicts chased him block after block, threatening to catch up and do him in. It was physically impossible to run far enough, fast enough, to outdistance the ghosts. Sooner or later, he would collapse; when he did, the ghosts would win. Fear creates what it fears. Just when it seems all will be lost, the Adult learns to cry for help.

The Concept of the Inner Child

As I stated in Chapter 4, I first became aware of the concept of the Inner Child of the Past in the writings of child psychiatrist Hugh Missildine. This writing came out in 1963, and I devoured it. It was the first time I understood the need to seek to understand myself and to process my own family-of-origin issues. Soon after this discovery, I studied with Tom Harris, who is the author of the book *I'm OK, You're OK* (1969) and based his writing on the work of Eric Berne and transactional analysis. From there I became part of the Transactional Analysis Association in San Francisco and continued to do research in this area. More recently, I discovered the writing of Charles Whitfield in *Healing the Child Within* (1989). I have given copies of this book to many counselees and have reread Whitfield several times myself. His workbook on healing the Inner Child is an excellent resource.

As per Whitfield's discussion, the Inner Child that develops during the presocial years of childhood can continue to play old tapes from early experiences of how to perceive self, life, significant others, God, and relationships. If not updated, these tapes foster plenty of delusions, fears, "malignant perceptions," and downright lies about who we are and what we are worth which cripple us when such feelings are allowed to control our thinking.

THE TYRANNY OF THE INNER CHILD

A Four-Year-Old Within Controls the Adult Outside

In other words, a four-year-old inside me can be telling me decades later how to perceive myself and my worth. What does that four-year-old know about present reality and who I really am? We encounter people along the walks of life who still live out those earlier perceptions as if they were the gospel truth. They are Adult Children who have not been set free from their painful pasts.

Dan, an adult, fully capable of living life responsibly, compassionately, lovingly, caringly, and honestly, came to a time of crisis when earlier fears and perceptions of failure began to surface. Instead of seeing those reactions for what they were—delusions from the past which emanate from within the Inner Child—he was caught off balance by their intensity. In that moment, Dan forgot who he was, what he had accomplished, that others truly love and understood him. Dan gave in to that Inner Child and reverted back to earlier childhood forms of thinking, which crippled him.

Know the Truth

Jesus Christ said, "and you will know the truth, and the truth will make you free" (John 8:32, RSV). The truth concerns the reality of who that little Child of the past is and what happened to him when his real needs went unmet and he thought it was because something was wrong with him. The truth also relates to who the Adult counterpart really is. The Adult Dan is a wonderful, unrepeatable creation of God, made to be loved and learning how to be loving. Nevertheless, this truth totally escaped the mixed-up Dan in crisis. That capable, compassionate Dan, a caring human being who is the apple of God's eye and is loved unconditionally and is worth Jesus Christ to God the Father, was lost in the maze of delusional feelings.

Even if Dan had failed in that classroom (which he did not), that does not mean he was a failure. Dan was not a failure when he could not straighten out his dysfunctional childhood family; he was not one when he made mistakes and things did not go right. Dan has never really been a failure—and this is the key—except in his *own* self-perceptions.

Little Dan did the only thing a kid can do: he let those significant others who failed him off the hook by blaming himself for the failures of his family of origin. Then he put that same garbage on himself when he reflected back on that classroom war zone. He could not see the bright light he reflected, the grace-filled influence he exerted, the good he did, the drops of blood he sweated for them and over them, nor could he see that they were facing *their* own failures, not his.

The Power of Past Delusions

These earlier delusions of the past are still in action, still in control. We make those delusions our reality; when we do that, they become our own self-imposed dungeon. There, we hide like beaten pups, imprisoned within our own self-perceptions, fearing we will never get free, while the door is unlocked for escape throughout. The barriers to freedom exist because of self-imposed delusions. We have done damage to ourselves.

In that classroom struggle, Dan held up a delusional, distorted mirror of the image he saw, which he thought was his true self. Dan saw reflected back the feelings of his childhood, and those fears and delusions and misconceptions seemed real. Believing them to be reality, Dan panicked and ran. If Diana, his wife, had not called for him to stop he might have kept running until he could not run anymore.

God's Rescue

Either way, God is out in front ready to catch His child when he finally collapses in faith and trust following a season of despair. God comes through many sources: a caring mate, a sensitive physician, a listening friend, or a moment of silence after the "wind, earthquake, and fire" (see 1 Kings 19:11-13). When God speaks, it is to the adult—that part of the human psyche that can reason and test reality and become self-aware. God does not speak to that archaic part of the ego structure, the Inner Child of the Past who cannot handle adulthood and adult responsibilities and adult perceptions.

God, the Holy Spirit, the Spirit of Truth, brings the insights of truth to the adult who lives in the present and can learn to predict the future and "love others as he loves himself." This is the Dan who is the pastor, social worker, and teacher, husband, father, and friend. If he is willing to allow the Inner Child of the Past to heal from those prejudices and delusions, then he can learn to respect the child of the past and be his friend. Nevertheless, the adult Dan must be in control. The adult Dan must be conscious of who he is so that this healthy level of self-awareness can lead to spontaneity and intimacy. Love is letting go of fear, as expressed in 1 John 4:18-21:

> There is no fear in love, but perfect love casts out fear. For fear has to do with punishment, and he who fears is not perfected in love. We love because he first loved us. If anyone says, "I love God," and hates his brother, he is a liar; for he who does not love his brother whom he has seen, cannot love God whom he has not seen. And this is the commandment we have from him, that he who loves God should love his brother also. (RSV)

The Adult Who Is Set Free

The Inner Child's fear of a lack of worth and capability and responsibility can be exchanged for the truth of his or her true worth and capability to love and be loved. When crisis comes, the freed-up adult, healed from the control of the delusions of the Inner Child, knows how to act and, if in doubt, whom to ask for help and assistance. The contaminated Adult is too easily influenced and/or controlled by the delusional Child. This contaminated Adult knows only how to surrender and allow the delusional Child to control life crises through panic, fear, and anxiety attacks. Consequently, the free adult, when faced with situations that are uncomfortable and threatening, knows what to do to get through crises in the best possible way.

Adult Children of Dysfunctional Pasts

The delusional Inner Child cannot handle such gravity of situation and will always panic and place blame and shame. What four-year-old can handle marriage, employment, or other difficulties or adult responsibilities? Yet, in reality, four-year-olds within adults drive cars and resort to road rage, walk out on their families, steal what they believe they have a right to, drop out of life and expect to be cared for no matter what, and carry on the dysfunctional lifestyles to which they grew accustomed from childhood. We call such people "Adult Children."

These are children living in the bodies of adults. They can disguise themselves as clinicians, doctors, lawyers, teachers, laborers, pastors, prophets, crusaders, or perpetual "kids." Inside such adults is an Inner Child of the Past who fears the relationships, the crises, the pressures, and the circumstances that overwhelm the Adult and who initiates the eruption that will let the world know for sure that herein lies a hurt, confused, pained, scared Child, totally out of control. Whenever the Inner Child is in control, the Adult on the outside is out of control (Farmer, 1990).

Outcomes for the Healing of the Inner Child

When the process of healing is well on its way, a responsible adult in charge emerges with a good level of self-awareness of who the *real* person is, what potential and gifts he or she has, and how to respond to life and the real needs of others in loving and caring ways.

Dan has been learning how to deal with little Dan—that Inner Child of the Past—through the recognition that little Dan is ever present and a valuable part of his total psyche. Nevertheless, little Dan was assuming a family role he could not fulfill as a child in the past or now as an Adult in the present. The Child could not cope with adult life. The Child's true role was to be a child when he was a child, despite the fact that he had been forced by circumstances to assume an "adult" stance as a child. The Child could never cope with adulthood, then or now.

Dan the adult has to be in control. This means Dan has to reconnect with little Dan. Adult Dan has to reparent himself—so little Dan will not seek to fulfill the antiquated role of "family rescuer." Little Dan then could be free to have the childhood he never had. Dan the adult would care for present relationships and responsibilities. Furthermore, when little Dan finds himself panicked by life, adult Dan can guide him through the darkness to victory and success. The panic attacks would no longer be needed. The adult is fully capable of handling—with God's help—anything that presents itself. If the adult needs help, he knows where to turn.

EGO STATES AND TRANSACTIONAL ANALYSIS

The Child Ego State

Three ego states exist, according to transactional analysis (Missildine, 1963; Berne, 1964; Harris, 1969). First is the Child Ego State, which develops from birth to about age five, the presocial years. Much of the worldview of the Child Ego State is based on delusional feelings acquired while relating to significant others. The experiences of the Child Ego State require the emerging Adult Ego State to process and reality-test them. In the absence of an emerging Adult Ego State, these delusions become the Child's Ego State reality.

The Parent Ego State

Parallel with the Child Ego State is the developing Parent Ego State, which also emerges between birth and age five. Much of the worldview encompassed in the emerging Parent Ego State is composed of prejudices gleaned from relating to the same significant others who care for the child in these emerging years between birth and age five. Without an emerging Adult Ego State to reality-test these prejudices, distortions can develop in the Parent Ego State's view of reality in the developing self. These prejudices extend to views of self, others, life, God, and the interpretation of life experiences.

The Adult Ego State

The saving factor is the development of the Adult Ego State at around ten to twelve months of age. Unless the development of the Adult Ego State is hindered by the Child and/or Parent Ego States, the Adult Ego State will continue to develop throughout one's life.

Everyone needs a capable Adult Ego State for reality testing, predicting, and understanding what it means to be "fully human, fully alive." The Adult Ego State also draws upon the positive inputs from the Inner Child and the Parent of the Self. Nevertheless, the Adult Ego State remains in control, leading the individual to awareness, spontaneity, and intimacy. By the time an individual is out of the parental home and on his or her own, he or she should be freed up so the Adult Ego State can be in charge and create relationships that are meaningful, open, flexible, and spontaneous. Such an individual possesses a much greater ability to love and be loved.

When the Child Ego State contaminates the Adult and keeps it bound to earlier delusions, the Adult appears to be more an "adult child" than a responsible, loving, caring, interdependent person. When the Parent Ego State contaminates the Adult, it keeps the Adult bound by prejudice, self-justification, blame, shame, and regret. When both Child and Parent Ego States are allowed in varying degrees to contaminate the Adult Ego State, self-blame, shame, perfectionism, fear, guilt, anxiety, and a whole range of negative emotions cripple the functioning of the person. These maladies, of course, can become extreme and are often expressed in many forms of mental illness (see Figure 5.1 on ego states). Those of us who did not choose our significant others very wisely have a lot of baggage to deal with if the Adult Ego State within us is contaminated by the Child and Parent Ego States and needs to be freed up.

RECOVERY

Healing for the Caregiver

In Dan's case and in my own, we assumed the roles of family rescuers and probably became counselors in our adult lives for that very reason. We must deal with this baggage of the past to find our own rescue and healing.

God, who is ultimate reality, deals with us in reality, and we need to be in reality with God to hear and respond to Him meaningfully. The Child and Parent Ego States will never suffice. These ego states are archaic. Life as it must be lived needs to be real and needs to be in the present. The freed-up Adult Ego State is the real thing.

The healing process—the reality testing—and the freeing up of the Adult is the work of the Holy Spirit. Hence, the Holy Spirit as the Spirit of Truth reveals to us and within us "the truth that sets us free" (John 8:32). This freedom is freedom from the delusions and prejudices that cripple us and keep us captive. The fruit of this freedom is the ability to love and be loved. That love not only includes loving the Triune God and others, but also oneself.

Few Inner Children were ever taught to love themselves. Few Inner Parents were ever given reasons to value themselves. Our dysfunctional beginnings taught us just the opposite, and we learned these negative lessons well. Now it is time to *unlearn* such bad lessons. Any learned responses can be unlearned, and the truth can be substituted in their place.

During our calls that August of 1999, I attempted to show Dan how God sees him, how I see him, and what a beautiful spiritual being he truly is. When he could perceive this, then the healing became measurable, fear lost its icy grip, and the anxiety lost its reason for being.

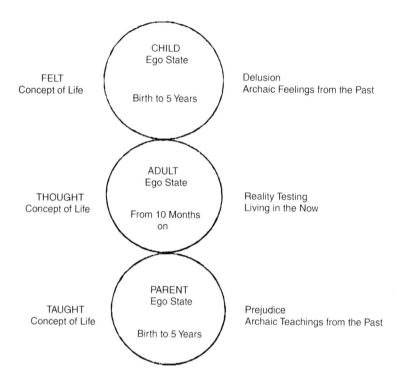

FIGURE 5.1. Transactional Analysis

The Child Ego State develops between birth and around five years, the presocial period. It gleans feelings from encounters with significant adults and older siblings out of which is formed a felt concept of life and the world surrounding the child. The Parent Ego State develops simultaneously out of the life lessons taught and caught within that environment. Many of the Child feelings are delusional and many of the lessons caught are prejudicial, but the small child is unable to make these kinds of judgments. The emerging Adult Ego State, which begins to develop around ten months of age and continues through life, learns to test the reality of feelings and thoughts and thus produces a rational thought concept of life. The Adult Ego State, once freed up from the control of the Child and Parent, is able to achieve awareness, spontaneity, and intimacy. It can also draw on the positive feelings of the Inner Child and the reality-tested lessons of the Inner Parent, and thus the Inner Adult learns to parent itself. The Adult is the part of the ego structure capable of decision making, problem solving, relationship building and maintaining, and becoming fully human. The Child and Parent are not capable of handling such realities; they stop developing around age five.

Even though one's healing process persists for a lifetime, healing can move ahead in leaps and bounds when the truth is realized.

Missildine (1963) helps us to identify what is the present by helping us to understand the results of earlier behavior patterns involving those significant others in our lives. Harris (1969) helps us to understand the mechanics of how ego states develop and solidify but can, nevertheless, change and yield to therapy and healing. Whitfield (1989) gives us considerable guidance for the healing process of the Inner Child and the concurrent pain. Powell (1976) helps us to discover the goals of true healing. Seamands (1981) leads us to the knowledge of how God is present in our healing. For those seriously traumatized by abuse in childhood, Farmer (1990) gives us a program of recovery worth considering. Finally, Wright (1985) shows us how we can truly make peace with our past.

Notwithstanding all we have just discussed, it is God who oversees the entire process. The writers cited help set the stage for healing, but it is God who heals. His Spirit bears witness with our spirit as to who we really are in Him. When we discover our true worth in Him, we overflow with love for Him; we love our significant others, those who need us, and even those who reject us—for we have learned to love others as we love ourselves. We are free to love and be loved.

We grew up believing that if someone—anyone—would just love us, then life might make sense. Nevertheless, we come to realize in our healing that even though it is important to be loved, the most important thing of all is *being able to love*. "He who loves knows God, for God is love" (1 John 4:7).

Chapter 6

How the Suffering of the Caregiver Benefits the Caregiver-Client Relationship—Part 1

Daniel Langford

The Corruption of Proverbs in Translation

Proverbs frequently suffer corruption in transmission. What happens is sort of like the party game Telephone. Players sit in a circle, and a message is relayed around the circle by being whispered in the ear of each player. When the message gets to the end, the last player says aloud the message he got, which is usually nothing like what was whispered by the first person. So it has been with the proverb of "walking in another man's moccasins." The proverb, attributed to an unidentified Native American, gets modified to fit whatever story is being told.

The Origin of the Native American Moccasin Proverb

I wanted to find out if this aphorism was really spoken by a Native American, so I did some digging. The research paid off, and though I did not find the name of a specific person, I found a Native American proverbs Web site (2000) that attributes the maxim to the Cheyenne nation. The correct rendering is as follows:

Do not judge your neighbor until you have walked two moons in his moccasins. (p. 2)

Hence, the application can logically be made from "judging" to "understanding." The Langford paraphrase reads like this:

> You cannot really understand the suffering another person experiences until you have lived that experience yourself.

The Significance of Communication, Understanding, and Empathy

Understanding implies communication and connection with the life of another person. John Powell (1976), whose book *Fully Human, Fully Alive* has provided much of the inspiration for this writing, states one of the insights that has changed his life: "The success or failure of human relationships is determined primarily by success or failure at communication" (p. 3). Consequently, our success in effectively relating to others not only as caregivers but as fellow human beings hinges on our ability to communicate with another person.

The Oxford English Dictionary (OED) (2000) defines the intransitive verb form of *communicate* as "To have a common part, take part, partake, participate, share . . . with (a person)." An additional nuance of meaning is found with this usage of the word:

> To hold intercourse or converse; (now always) to impart, transmit, or exchange thought or information (by speech, writing, or signs) . . . to convey one's thoughts, feelings, etc., successfully; to gain understanding or sympathy. (p. 4)

Thus, to communicate implies participation in the life of another to the point that one shares not only words but the experiences of that individual in a deeper way other than mere assent to the surface of conversation. This brings us to the concept of empathy, which has kinship to *communication* and to *understanding*.

The OED (2000) defines empathy as follows: "The power of projecting one's personality into (and so fully comprehending) the object of contemplation" (p. 1).

So here we have kindred words joined together in a sort of linguistic, molecular bond:

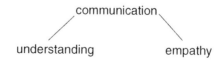

communication

understanding   empathy

This bonding of words implies that the real connection between one individual and another goes beyond the mere sharing of information. Understanding is more than denotations of words and phrases. Communication is more than saying, "Yes, I hear you talking, and I recognize the words you are using." The whole is greater than the sum of its parts: real communication and real understanding involve the projection of our own being (personality) and experiences into the experiences of the one we desire to communicate with. The result, as the interacting definitions imply, is that we share self with another self: we become fellow travelers walking down the road of life, partaking of the same chalice of experiences. True communication/empathy/understanding incorporates or brings together two lives to share the same insights and feelings.

The OED also defines *communicate* as uniting in the observance of Communion or the Lord's Supper. The symbolic tie to the above analogy is powerful. Liturgical churches equate communion as the partaking of the body and blood of Jesus Christ, symbolized in the receiving of bread and wine. Hence, the body and blood of Christ are ingested in us, and those elements in a spiritual way become part of us. We know Christ because we have eaten his flesh and drunk his blood (John 6:53, NIV). This Christianized use of *communicate* adds extraordinary significance to the term in our relationship with others: we partake in another's life to the point that we share experiences with that person from a mutual frame of reference.

The Importance of Boundaries

I am not proposing that real understanding/communication/empathy means that we sacrifice personal identity or our own sense of self. Our self remains intact. It is just that we go beyond the comfortable circle of our own image of the world and attempt to partake in the experiences of another human being for whatever reason—to be a friend or to provide care. We can do neither if we refuse to come down from our insulated ivory tower.

Carl Rogers and Empathy

Carl Rogers, intriguingly, came to the same conclusions that I did. Rogers (1961) contends that to be effective with someone you are attempting to help, the caregiver has to understand the feelings of the client and accept those feelings without minimizing, judging, or presenting any moral or diagnostic evaluation. In essence, the caregiver is a companion to the client and walks by his or her side.

Rogers explains that this relationship is not achieved by the therapist disconnecting himself or herself from the client. Rogers sees true progress as being accomplished if he, as the therapist, is open with the client regarding his own experiences, which in turn gives the client freedom to be open with his or her own experiences.

The Mutual Experience of Suffering Creates a Special Bond Between People

This, then, is an advantage to have when working with someone in need. If you have known suffering, and the person who comes to you is experiencing suffering—and if, per chance, his or her suffering is very similar to an experience you have gone through—you, as the caregiver, have the unique opportunity to share a client's pain with an understanding that someone who has not gone through the experience could ever fully appreciate.

Here is an example. I shared the story of my panic attacks with a non-blood relative in my extended family. I remember that as I told my story, this person found the freedom to open up, cry, and express the deep feelings of pain regarding her own struggle with panic. This relative's daughter wanted to hear more because panic issues were a part of her extended family. Healing and hope were generated in this special moment. My experience with panic allowed these other people to feel free to express their experiences with panic—and just that alone. Being with someone else who knows how it feels was a healing moment for everyone, including the messenger. No profound or erudite lecture was given; it was just people sharing life. The crowning moment of this special time occurred after a break in the conversation (which was at a family gathering) when one of them left for a moment and then returned. Putting her hand on my shoulder, she said, "Thank you." No other words were needed. She knew I understood her pain.

The Futility of Teaching or Lecturing to Make a Person Well

Rogers points out that teaching or lecturing a person to make them well is an effort in futility. He concludes from his experience with clients that he cannot help a "troubled person" by means of "intellectual or training procedures." He believes that these approaches are futile and elicit only a temporary change that "soon disappears" and leaves the person feeling intensely inadequate (pp. 32-33).

Power That Comes When the Caregiver Has a Repertoire of Experience As a Patient

The caregiver becomes the patient; the caregiver needs help; the caregiver faces his own vulnerability and, as a result, the caregiver becomes a more powerful, albeit wounded, healer because he or she can offer firsthand experience about what it is like to hurt rather than just spout off technical babble from a manual that gives the sterile facts of a disorder without the connection of empathy. All of this reflection brings us to a theological crossroads where these principles were taught over 1900 years ago.

The Bible and the Benefit of Suffering

Second Corinthians 1:3-4 is the paean or hymn of praise for the wounded healer. The words of rejoicing read this way:

> Praise be to the God and Father of our Lord Jesus Christ, the Father of compassion and the God of all comfort, who comforts us in all our troubles, so that we can comfort those in any trouble with the comfort we ourselves have received from God. (NIV)

Suffering, healing, and sharing the fragility of our life experiences with another human being are the ingredients for powerful involvement with someone who is in trouble.

William Barclay (1975b) comments on this passage as follows:

> The supreme result of all this is that we gain the power to comfort others who are going through it. Paul claims that the things which have happened to him and the comfort which he has re-

ceived have made him able to be a source of comfort to others. Barrie tells how his mother lost her dearest, and then he says, "That is where my mother got her soft eyes and why other mothers ran to her when they had lost a child." . . . It is worth while experiencing suffering and sorrow if that experience will enable us to help others struggling with life's billows. (p. 171)

A Crucible of Adversity with Unexpected Outcomes

Another example of how adversity helped me to provide comfort in a very unexpected way happened over nine years ago. My family and I were in a very difficult crossroads in our lives. At the time, I was pastoring a small church, and we made a decision to change the locale of our ministry by seeking to start a new church in a desert community of Southern California—a sort of leap of faith. For many reasons, these plans fell apart, and we were sidelined and took up residence in the home of Diana's mother in Rocklin, California. We were homeless refugees of dreams gone awry. While we were in this limbo in Rocklin, we attempted to restart a bookstore and office supply business that had sustained us when we were pastoring on California's north coast. Despite our best efforts, this venture fell apart as well. We were at a very low point because of two distressing life events.

Though these experiences at the time seemed very difficult to understand, the pain we endured provided new insights and new opportunities for growth. It goes back again to the Cheyenne story of the moccasins. When you are walking in another person's shoes of adversity, you develop a compassion, an empathy for such a person's distress that you could not have had before.

In my case, the painful road of collapsed dreams and financial travails helped me to develop a deep appreciation for the poor and those going through recovery from addictions that had devastated their lives. Consequently, unexpected opportunities to support others as well as experience personal revitalization unfolded as a result of enduring these troubles.

I told part of this story in an article that came out in *Decision* magazine in February 1994. The following excerpt recounts what happened when I accepted a position as a chaplain at an alcohol and drug recovery hospital following the failure of our business. The setting was an institutional AA (Alcoholics Anonymous) meeting that I attended as part of my duties.

> One day, as I listened to stories of addictions and struggles toward recovery, my mind, darkened by grief, was suddenly illuminated with fresh insight. Here I was, a minister to recovering alcoholics, yet in reality I was in need of recovery just as they were. My life too had become unmanageable. They and I were not that different from one another; we were as one in our sufferings and in the challenge of recovery.
>
> My eyes brimmed with tears when it was my turn to speak. I looked intently at each participant as I said, "I have a story too. My problem is not drinking, but I have agonized just as you have. My business failed; I lost thousands of dollars; my family has suffered; I feel hopeless, and I too need recovery."
>
> They understood. We embraced, for we had discovered that we were as one. "The God of all comfort" was there for me in an unexpected way in that unexpected place. (Langford, 1994, p. 32)*

The above story echoes what Carl Rogers (1961) said about transparency. When I transparently share who I am with others and accept others for who they are, "I become a companion to my client, accompanying him in a frightening search for himself, which he now feels free to undertake" (p. 34).

Nevertheless, the opportunity to become a companion (a fellow traveler) to recovering alcoholics was not the only unexpected point of contact with others who needed a companion. The article in *Decision* circulated around the world via 1,000,000 copies. One of those readers, who lived in Ohio, phoned me about six months after that issue of the magazine was published.

The evening I received this phone call followed a very stressful day. When I answered the phone, I was in a grumpy mood. The unfamiliar voice of the caller asked for me, and I abruptly replied, "Listen! If you are a telemarketer, I have had a busy day, and I do not want to talk to you."

The caller replied, "No, I am not a telemarketer. I read your story in *Decision* magazine, and your experience is just like mine. What you wrote encouraged me very much, and I just wanted to say thank you."

---

*This article was taken from *Decision* magazine, February, 1994; ©1994 Billy Graham Evangelistic Association, used by permission, all rights reserved.

I was abashed by my curt manner. I apologized for being inconsiderate, and this gentleman and I shared for a brief moment the agonies of our mutual losses and the comfort of communicating as fellow sufferers of misfortune. A healing occurred for both of us because we had been down the same road.

Experiences, Good or Bad, Change Us

Robert Schuller (1982) once said that events good or bad change us, and we are never the same after we go through those events. The same is true about the relationship between a caregiver and his or her client. The client is not the only one to benefit or change; the caregiver benefits and changes as well. The relationship between the client and the therapist is mutually beneficial, and each learns from the other with the result that the therapist and the client become more fully "actualized" as an outcome of their encounter with each other.

As I said earlier, my losses and subsequent recovery gave me a deeper appreciation for the sufferings of the poor and those whose lives have been devastated by addictions. Because of this deeper appreciation of these human sufferings, my interest was kindled in becoming a more effective helper. So an additional positive outcome of some very negative experiences was my acceptance into a social work master's program at California State University in Sacramento. I graduated in 1996 with an MSW (master's in social work) and with additional expertise to make a difference in the lives of those who need encouragement and a helping hand. All of these experiences of good fortune came out of a crucible of adversity, loss, and grief which at the time appeared to make no sense.

Aseity and Issues of Transference

I realize that two of the objections that can be raised regarding the previous discussion are role reversals of the client and therapist and issues of transference—that is, the danger of the therapist projecting his life problems upon the client and the hazard of the therapist using the client to meet his or her own needs. Please let me clarify that none of this discussion about sharing in suffering is intended to advocate a style of caregiving that reverses the role of the therapist with the client in inappropriate or exploitive ways.

Boundaries and Differentiation

The keys to avoiding transference and role reversal are *boundaries* and *differentiation*. Emil Authelet will explore these issues comprehensively in Chapter 7. Nevertheless, the mutuality of experience with another does not mean that we become that other person who shares our experience. Rogers (1961) particularly emphasizes the otherness and separateness of the client (p. 34). Hence, being a companion and sharing vulnerability with someone else does not mean we violate the boundaries of that person or of ourselves.

Friedman (1985) offers insight when he discusses family dynamics and the relationship between clergy and their congregations. Citing the work of Murray Bowen of Georgetown Medical School, Friedman suggests the following:

> What Bowen has hypothesized is a scale of differentiation. Differentiation means the capacity of a family member to define his or her own life goals apart from the surrounding togetherness pressures, to say "I" when others are demanding "you" and "we." . . . The concept should not be confused with autonomy or narcissism, however. Differentiation means the capacity to be an "I" while remaining connected. (p. 27)

The key phrase is the last one: "to be an 'I' while remaining connected." This combination of relational qualities is frequently missing in the interaction between a caregiver and the person he or she is trying to help, and, typically, it is not the loss of the therapists' boundaries of self as it is the failure to establish a genuine connection with the client as described by Carl Rogers.

Empathy versus Aseity

Reconsidering the positive points of appropriate and empathic connection between a therapist and client, I do not know if the habit of some counselors of distancing themselves or disconnecting from the client is a relic from the psychoanalytic approach. Nonetheless, I would argue that treatment that is not built upon mutual respect, two-way communication, and a nonhierarchical relationship between the client and therapist means that everyone loses. The person being helped fails to discover the common bonds of human vulnerability that he or she shares with the caregiver, and the caregiver fails to develop a therapeutic environment in which the person being helped has the freedom to express deep life issues without the fear of condemnation. We as human beings are on a level playing field when it comes to the pageant of life. We arrive in the same way and we go out the same way. The existential determinants of uncontrolled birth and inevitable death are shared by all humans. Hence, our mission as caregivers is to learn how to make the life that exists between the curtains of birth and death most meaningful and fulfilling to ourselves and those we have been called to help who cross our paths. This cannot be done in an ivory tower of professional aseity.

Some Final Thoughts

I am not suggesting that a caregiver necessarily must experience everything that the patient or client is going through in order to help that person. But I am saying that the repertory of experiences we gain in our own struggles with life and growth have empathic power if we can use this part of our "self" to attempt to understand what the other person who has come to us for help is experiencing.

True, the physician who has never had cancer does not have to get cancer to effectively treat a cancer patient. Nonetheless, if such a physician has experienced cancer and treats a cancer patient, each has a deep understanding that those without the experience cannot really share.

This brings up another point. None of us has been called to rescue the world. There are people we cannot help because it is not our mission to help everyone. Rogers (1961) affirmed as much when he said, "I am by no means always able to achieve this kind of relationship with another, and sometimes, even when I feel I have achieved it in myself, he may be too frightened to perceive what is offered to him" (p. 35).

Consequently, we are going to be more effective with some than with others simply because (once again) we have walked similar paths. Those who have walked down paths similar to our own are special people to whom we as caregivers have been commissioned to offer our care. Others walking down different paths and sharing a different set of experiences will be commissioned to serve those people whom we could not help effectively from our repertory of experiences. This is okay.

At the heart of the caregiver's mission are two words, *therapy* and *comforter.* The word *therapy* has a Greek etymological root, *therapeo,* which means healing. Concurrently, *comforter* is rooted in the Greek word *parakleetos,* which means one who is called to the aid of or to stand beside another (Arndt and Gingrich, 1979). What more fitting description is there of a caregiver when you combine the Greek origins of comfort and therapy:

> Caregiver: an agent of healing who comes to aid and stand beside the person he or she serves as an advocate, encourager, and companion.

Chapter 7

How the Suffering of the Caregiver Benefits the Caregiver-Client Relationship—Part 2

Emil Authelet

INTRODUCTION

Each of us lives life from the inside out. We may act or react to the external world, but how we act or react is determined by what is inside. As Jesus taught, it is out of the heart that life's issues flow (Matthew 15:18). We live out what is inside of us.

The Suffering of the Caregiver Brings Out the Authentic Person from Within

The caregiver is first of all a person who is trained and equipped to offer care and to bring to the therapeutic relationship who he or she is. Furthermore, the therapist is a person who is also going through the process of becoming a fully developed human being. Consequently, the therapist extends his or her developing self for the benefit of the client/patient as the therapist himself or herself reaches out to the fulfillment of the person he or she is becoming.

Another aspect of this is the life journey of the caregiver and especially the levels of personal suffering the caregiver has experienced and how these levels have impacted his or her life's journey. As a result of these life experiences, changes take place within the caregiver that can enhance or hinder the person's abilities to offer care. These experiences have the ability to give back one's true self, refined and matured, or can leave the caregiver self-focused, struggling, and ingrown. In being tested by life, we go through the fires of personal sorrows and suffering and, as a result, life offers back to us our enhanced true selves if we are open to such growth. It is out of our true selves that we become better caregivers. In the process, we discover who we really are, and this prepares us for being our best in service to others.

We Give Back to Others What We Have Learned in Our Own Struggle for Survival

We cannot offer to others what we ourselves have never experienced and, therefore, our own healing through suffering is what we speak out of and what makes us the caregivers we are becoming. We are, on one hand, caregivers in spite of our own sufferings and, on the other hand, we are caregivers because of our own sufferings and the skills we acquired to overcome those sufferings.

Dan was a caregiver before his own crisis in 1999; he is now the caregiver he could never have been without the growth process provided in and through his own personal crisis. What we do as caregivers flows from what is inside us. We share out of who we are; we relate out of what we have become and are becoming.

Unresolved Issues of the Therapist Can Harm the Client

Unease within us as caregivers leads to disservice to the client. So a caregiver who has never dealt with his or her own issues, is doing the client a real disservice. Accordingly, what is needed is not something from a textbook or a series of workshops; what is needed is a genuine sharing of person with person. It usually takes a crisis to get us to do this depth work. The person of the caregiver is interacting with the person of the client; the magic that occurs between them is the therapeutic relationship leading to healing within both persons.

Requirements for Effective Caregiving

This is what is required if the caregiver is to relate objectively (as much as possible) to the client so that the needs of the client, not those of the therapist, are the main focus. Therapist and client give to each other in the transaction. However, the primary focus is on the needs of the client. When Dan called in the middle of the night, he needed someone to listen to him, not someone to talk at him. Dan needed to be heard and helped, not used or held at arm's length. Dan needed someone who could empathize with his pain and fright—someone who could hear where he was coming from and meet him there. What he wanted most was to hear, "I hear you," followed by "I understand," and hopefully, in time, "I've been there and here's what worked for me." The dark tunnel has been walked by others, and the light at the end is really there. Hope lies ahead and "We can walk the road together."

The Arena of the Caregiver

Caregivers work mainly with hurting persons who have experienced varying levels of trauma, pain, alienation, and emotional crisis. A caregiver does not have to have experienced a similar level of pain to empathize with the pain of the client. However, a caregiver who has never dealt meaningfully with the levels of his or her own pain brings the failure to address personal issues into the therapeutic relationship. All attempts at objectivity aside, this failure does interfere with the ability to relate between the therapist and client and, consequently, a bias against healing is put in place. The client should not have to find healing despite the therapist; the opposite should be true.

The therapist should be far enough along in his or her own process to be able to meet the client where he or she is and assist him or her to recover and grow. The therapist should convey, in essence, "This is what worked for me, and I know it can help you in finding your own healing" (Schaef, 1992, 1998).

A Friend's Loss

A friend of mine lost his wife to cancer recently. It has been a terrible blow for him, and he is well aware of the fact that it has shaken the very foundations of his life and thinking. This friend, when he has taken the time needed to do his grief work and has been allowed time to heal and reaffirm his foundational beliefs about himself, God, and life, will be a very different therapist than he was when his wife was still alive and they were happily engaged in a vibrant relationship they believed would last for decades more. The depth of his pain in his loss will mark the depth of his new growth as a person and, thus, as a professional caregiver. His ability to resonate with the pain within another will be greatly enhanced. We grow through crisis and suffering. These are the elements that mature us.[1]

WHAT MAKES A GOOD CAREGIVER?

A Christian view of caregiving, based upon a Christian worldview and commitment to persons in need, seeks to fulfill the command of Jesus as given in John 13, "Love one another, as I have loved you" (Haugk, 1984; Haugk and McKay, 1994).[2] This gets worked out in the following ways:

1. The ability to accept where the client is coming from without judgment and to meet him or her there. This level of honest acceptance then leads to an understanding of where he or she needs to be within a moral framework that leads to healing, wholeness, and full living as a responsible, loving, caring spiritual being.
2. To respond with empathy, not sympathy or identification. To be able to enter others' pain and understand their trauma and to help lead them through it without making it one's own or drowning with them in it.
3. Acquiring the ability to feel the pain of another, yet to understand it is the client's pain and not one's own. "This is your pain; I now know how this has affected you. Let's explore options you may have for dealing with it."
4. Listening to learn and know how to care, never assuming one knows the real need until discerned through relating with the client. "Help me understand how you perceive it and how it is affecting your life and thinking."
5. The ability to hear what is really there and why; to get beyond the presenting need to the real need. The skill to get to the underlying cause and effect and to assist the client in seeing things as they really are.
6. Resonating without identifying and then responding appropriately to what is really being heard: "This is what I hear you saying; this is how it has affected you. This is what you are struggling with."
7. Above all else, this question arises for the skilled active listener: "Am I reading it right? Help me understand if you sense I am not with you."
8. A willingness to build and maintain a therapeutic relationship with the client: "Thank you for trusting me by sharing your

pain. Thank you for letting me work with you in your healing."

9. A willingness to extend the self for the well-being of the other: "It's important to me that you find the healing you need. We're working on this together."

10. To relate dependably as long as needed: "Our goal is your full healing. You will know when you have reached that goal."

11. To refer when necessary. "If I believe you need someone more skilled, I will help you find the person you need. If you feel you cannot share as needed with me, then I want you to let me know."

12. To work only for the well-being of the other. "My commitment to you is to work at my best for your well-being. We will evaluate how things are going from time to time."

13. To know how to establish and maintain healthy boundaries with the client. "In between sessions, if the need arises, here's how you may reach me."

14. To know how to care for oneself throughout the process. "My days off are these. I do take emergency calls at home if needed. By an emergency I mean this. . . ."

15. To maintain a good level of objectivity throughout the process. "My job is to challenge any perceptions I believe need to be reality-tested and to help you in your healing process. If you disagree, I ask only that you reflect on what we have shared together to see if anything changes within your perceptions. Your decision is final."

16. To help establish the conditions needed for healing. "Here is what I believe is needed for healing to take place. Let's commit to the process that will bring this about."

17. To allow God to do the healing. "God is the true Healer of all of life's hurts. My job is to help set the conditions so that healing can take place."

18. To celebrate the healing and allow the client to move forward in his or her process. "Now you are at a place where you can continue the process on your own. I'm here if you need help or to clarify something. I want you to know I am proud of you and the work you have done. All of Heaven rejoices, as do I!"

Why the Therapist-Client Relationship Is So Important

Taking clues from how Jesus related to those to whom He ministered through His healing presence, the following elements stand out:

1. True empathy is based within and communicated by the relationship being built and maintained between client and therapist. How this relationship is built and maintained determines the depth of the healing to take place. Healing occurs within the relationship.
2. The relationship is essential to the healing process. It does not happen apart from the relationship. If one could be healed by reading a book on healing, we would all be healed.
3. Interconnectedness is the key to the healing process working. The lack of interconnectedness led to the alienation in the first place. The therapeutic relationship may be the first genuine encounter within the client's life.
4. Illustration of Mark 1 and Jesus' encounter with a leper. He touched the leper before the healing took place because the deeper need was for human touch and loving or caring. The inner need was greater than the physical one (Mark 1:40-45).
5. The need for human touch. The Inner Child responds to touch more than anything else. When it has been missing the Child becomes crippled and confused. Healing of the total person includes the Child Ego State as well. This ego state is the key to healing. All feeling is within the Child.
6. The need has been created by faulty or dysfunctional relationships. Touch is the key to a Child's understanding of love and being loved. When it has been missing or in meager supply, distorted thinking and perception results.
7. Alienation is the root problem; reconciliation is the goal of the process. This happens while relating within the healing process.
8. The healing occurs within the relationship. The client comes to understand what went wrong before and what is right now in terms of holistic relating. The therapist offers acceptance, approval, and affirmation.
9. Caring is at work here. How the therapist cares for and about the client allows him or her to experience unconditional love and acceptance.

10. It gives the client something real to encounter and to reality test. Only the truth sets us free. This is how all significant relationships are to be.
11. The therapist is responsive, feeling, and committed. The client can trust the relationship, feel secure within it, and test holistic ways of relating within it.
12. The therapist and client interact. The client learns to be loved and to love. The client learns her or his gifts are valuable and worthwhile. He or she also learns how to succeed in relating meaningfully.

WE LIVE LIFE AND HELP OTHERS FROM THE INSIDE OUT

As God's spirit works with our spirit, so our spirit works with that of the person being helped. The healing takes place within that person's spirit and mind as a result of the encounter. The change from within the client dictates the healing. God does the healing; this is its locale.

1. The pain comes from within the client's life experience and the fears generated by these negative experiences. Getting down inside the client with acceptance and unconditional love allows the client to heal inside out.
2. The client's pain may resonate with the life experience of the therapist. The therapist, in tune with his or her own pain from the past, resonates with what is being presented by the client. We are one; we understand one another.
3. The client invites the therapist inside his or her issues. The trust level between them allows the client to share the full load with the therapist, knowing it is part of the healing process.
4. A relationship of mutual respect and trust is established. The therapist learns to trust the client's self-exposure. The client learns to trust the therapist's responses, insights, "care-frontations," and prodding.
5. To help in the healing process, one enters that pain empathetically. Being allowed into another's pain is a sacred trust and a powerful responsibility. Having been wounded yourself, you are

caringly sensitive to the wounds of another. The therapist enters to promote the client's healing and never to do harm.

6. Spirit responds to spirit; feelings are explored and shared. The emotional bridge between therapist and client is easily and often crossed as the process unfolds. With the sharing comes healing.

7. The therapist responds appropriately for the well-being of the client. Sensing what is truly needed by the client establishes the nature of the relating. The only agenda is the client's well-being.

8. The therapist responds out of who he or she is and knows. We share who we are as well as what we know. This makes for a genuine encounter the client can trust.

9. The healing takes place within the caring relationship. God, as the first party to the relationship, uses it to bring healing. Together we give the gift of love to the client.

10. The relationship is essential to the healing; healing takes place within the relating. But the goal does not end when the client believes he or she is loved but rather when the client is enabled to become loving and shares it with another.

11. The healing is within the relating. Healing cannot take place apart from a healing relationship.

12. The healing results in the client's ability to love and be loved. This is how we know healing has taken place.

Some Lessons Are Taught, Some Caught, and Others Experienced

The training of the therapist is essential.

1. The therapist's perceptions of reality are essential. These are what the client must encounter to heal. Thus, the faith, character, morality, and worldview of the therapist are also essential.

2. The life experiences of the therapist are essential. How the past has been handled and worked through is essential to the process. The ongoing healing of the therapist is a major factor in what the client is being offered.

3. The healing within the therapist is essential. It is out of this experience that the therapist speaks and relates.

4. The therapist is in process and is a part of the client's process. The therapist continues to heal and is able to speak out of major gains already experienced. Both therapist and client move toward the goal of maximum healing.
5. The process is shared between them. They are moving ahead together; both are in process. They share a common journey.
6. The process involves healing. No issue is inconsequential in the relationship. Little healings are also needed along the way. Big hurts need big healings; little hurts need healing, too.
7. The therapist models healing in the process. This is what it is like to find healing of one's past. This is what it is like to become fully human, fully alive.

The Jesus Way—Our Example

1. His understanding of the human condition. His empathy and compassion led Him to identify with human need and to fulfill it. He knows the human heart, mind, and will. He is able to offer total healing out of His wholeness.
2. His experiencing of the human condition is complete except for sinning. Being tempted in all points such as we, but without yielding to temptations, He becomes our example and our hope (Hebrews 4:15). He offers us His life and His healing. We have His forgiveness as well.
3. Being one with us experientially. He enters our pain and resolves it. He meets our deepest need and gives us His unconditional love and acceptance. We are made anew in Him and by Him. "The old has gone; the new has come" (2 Corinthians 5:17, NIV).
4. Knowing the real need beyond the presenting need, He invites us into wholeness within Himself. Once we experience that wholeness, then we are free to share it with others in His name.
5. Speaking from the answer and not the problem. Regardless of the problem, we have the answer in Him. The process of discerning the problem is individual; the solution to the problem is universal in the spiritual empowerment of Christ. He is the answer.

Boundary Issues Within the Therapeutic Relationship

1. Boundary issues within the therapeutic relationship are based on the needs of the client versus those of the therapist. The unmet needs of the therapist must not be allowed to affect the process. The need for wellness within the therapist is essential.
2. The needs of the client versus those of the therapist: the ability to enter into the needs of the client without becoming a part of them is essential. The process is taking place for the well-being of the client.
3. Maintain a high degree of objectivity. This requires more than skill on the part of the therapist. It also involves having dealt with one's own issues to allow for objectivity in relating to the client's issues.
4. Assisting another to face and move through his or her pain, having dealt with one's own pain first. Again, the concept of the "wounded healer" presupposes being able to assist the client with the process of healing experienced by the healer himself or herself.

The Grace of Walking in the Moccasins of Another Experiencing Suffering

1. The common bonds of our humanness: therapist and client meet as equals—one in the flesh; our experiences may differ but only in degree.
2. Knowing experientially and being able to share a commonness, a commonality. "Having been able to work through my own issues, I can patiently assist you in your dealing with yours. My growth encourages yours; yours encourages mine."
3. The therapist says, "I know what you are experiencing because I have been there. I know there is an answer. I am here for you, to journey with you into your discovery and healing."
4. The therapist continues: "This is what worked for me and why. It has also worked for others. You are unique, but your journey is not. You are a part of a whole, and your healing restores you to that whole."
5. Supportive statements can clarify the therapist's willingness to help and be present for the whole process: "I hear you." "I understand." "Let me help you with your pain." "I am here for

you." "No matter what you need to feel to heal, I am here to accompany you." "You can count on me being here for you."

A Fresh Look at Person-Centered Therapy

1. Reflecting back based on having entered into therapy. The client and therapist are making this journey together with God. Looking back for clarification and understanding, the pain can be re-entered and understood, seen for what it is, and moved beyond.
2. Knowing and feeling with another. Healing occurs within the redemptive relationship. The discovery of the truth sets the client free. New growth can now occur.
3. Becoming as one for the purpose of understanding and helping. The therapist is with the client through the client's pain and he or she sees it if for what it really was, free of distortion and delusion. This is freeing.
4. Entering into as an equal. One may be the therapist, and the other the client. However, they are equals. The client is experiencing unconditional love.
5. Healing comes from within. Just as the hurt was within, so is the healing. The important things are the healing of the hurt, the removal of the pain, and the establishing of a love relationship.

Spiritual Models of Caregiver Suffering and the Formation of the Wounded Healer

1. "Because I have been there, I can witness to the journey. I can serve as a guide. I can help you find the way for yourself."
2. "This is what has worked for me. When I was forced to make that journey, this is what happened within me and for me. This can be your experience as well."
3. Understanding one's own "woundedness" and healing process. "This is what my own woundedness meant to me and this is how it affected me. Is this how it affected you?"
4. The therapeutic process for therapist and client. "This is what I learned while going through my own process. This is what I would want for you to experience. As a result of this process, this is what we can be and become."

5. The I-Thou relationship and our mutual healing: "Just as a universal pool of pain exists that each takes from, so exists a universal center of healing we must tap. That source is God, and He is here to engulf us both in His process of healing."

How This Comes Together and Why

1. The healing process of the therapist flows with the healing process of the client. "What I have experienced is what I share with you. It has proven itself in my own journey toward healing."
2. The healing process of the client flows to the healing process of the therapist. "What you have experienced and are now experiencing you share with me, and together we test out its validity and impact."
3. The merging affirms the healing of both. "Our relating affirms the healing is taking place and you are learning to live at a new level of awareness and sharing. You are learning who you are, what you have to share, and how good it feels to be achieving wholeness."
4. The process assists the maturing of both. "Within our relationship we are both growing toward God, each other, our true selves, and others as well as toward life itself."
5. All healing is of God, who flows both to the therapist and the client. "He is the Source, and we are resourcing each other throughout the process He has ordained us in His grace and love."

THE CRITICAL ELEMENTS
OF THE HEALING PROCESS

1. God as the caregiver. "Our healing means more to Him than it ever could mean to us. He gives Himself to us for our healing. He is in it."
2. The caregiving of the therapist. "What I share with you is what God has shared with me. He has invited me to partner with Him in your healing."
3. The receiving of care by the client. "What you receive in and through this process is a direct gift from God. I am His partner in the process, but the result is of Him."

4. The process involving all three: "The divine triangle is God, you, and me. Each is active within the process. As the source of all healing, God is to be the focal point."
5. The resultant healing within the client and therapist. As the recipient of grace, and as the agent of grace, both are partaking of the divine source of grace—God.

When the Caregiver Fails to Deal with His or Her Own Issues

1. The level of caregiving extended to the client is less than needed. The level of sharing of oneself within the process determines the depth of the outcome. Both head and heart are required if the relationship is to be truly useful.
2. The inability to enter into the client's real needs. Unresolved issues within the therapist limit what can be offered. "My unresolved family-of-origin issues get in the way of being objective in assisting another with his or her issues."
3. When distance is felt, the client is confused and trust is hindered. How can one lead where one is afraid to go?
4. The caregiver's issues get in the way. It is time to refer and the client needs to know why. To continue at this point is to act dishonestly. The focus must be the real needs of the client.
5. Healing may or may not be possible for the client or the therapist. To act dishonestly is to rob the client. To act dishonestly has also indicated unmet needs within the therapist.

THE MEASURES OF A THERAPIST'S INTEGRITY AND SUCCESS

1. "I am a caregiver because . . . and I am aware of why. *My* therapist and I have explored this together. I am here to share my own healing."
2. "I have seen these results from my caregiving and they affirm how I am able to assist others in their healing. I am always in awe of the process, how it works, and its results within the client and myself."
3. "In caregiving, the quality of the relationship that is built between the client and me is of great importance to me. Meaningful

boundaries are essential. My focus must be on the well-being of the client."

4. "My perception of the client is that we are equals who are equally dependent upon God for healing, and we are in a relationship that may enhance or hinder the process. My genuine caring for and honest sharing with the client are essential elements to the success of this process."

5. "My perception of my role is that of partnering with God; in this partnering, I am using all the skills I have learned and give them to my client in order to give the gift of love to the recipient of my care."

CONCLUSION

1. "The healing arises from within the client and not from within me. What God shares with me is passed along to the client. The client learns to trust me just as I learn to trust God."

2. The therapist assists in the healing process. "Like a psychological, emotional midwife, new life is being created within the client, and I assist in this life being birthed."

3. All healing is of God. Only God can remedy alienation within and between persons. He alone can bring about forgiveness and new life. His unconditional love and grace are His healing agents.

4. The wounded healer is used in the process. "Not because I am whole, but because I have become aware of my woundedness and am willing to trust it to God for the healing only He can give. I am not yet whole; I am in the process of becoming."

5. Healing is shared by all within the process. To enter the process of healing for another benefit is to find new levels for oneself. To enter the process is to enter healing. To be in the process is to continually be maturing.

6. The truth has made us free. To learn the truth of who God is, who we are, who others are, and what life is all about is true freedom. It is to live in reality rather than in sin, delusion, and distortion.

7. We are free, indeed. The Inner Child and Parent are under the control of the free Adult. Potential exists for a growing aware-

ness, spontaneity, and intimacy. We are freed to love and be loved.

8. Healing is never complete; the process goes on and is shared. But the focus is on the present, with assurances of future growth and love. We are in harmony with God, others, self, and life. Life becomes more and more beautiful.

Chapter 8

Toward a Fresh Model of the Caregiver-Client Relationship: The Oneness of Human Experience—Part 1

Daniel Langford

INTRODUCTION

Vulnerability Is a Universal Human Condition

This chapter builds upon the discussion in Chapters 6 and 7 that emphasized the importance of a caregiver learning by walking along another's path in his or her moccasins so as to understand the pain and struggle that the client experiences. However, the focus for this chapter will be on the caregiver's own path and coming to terms with susceptibility to the vicissitudes of human experience that the caregiver shares with his client or patient.

I have come to accept in my own experience that I do not have to hide from others the frailty that exists in my being. I don't have to hide my story about panic attacks because, as we discussed in Chapters 6 and 7, such disclosure gives the freedom to others to open up without fear and say, "Hey! That is my problem, too! Here's my story."

I believe that as professionals in helping careers we do a disservice to those we are called to assist if we communicate the idea that "We've got it together. The reason that you, the clients, are coming to see us is that you don't have it together." Nothing could be further from the truth. Granted, I, as a therapist, may not share to the same degree the problems a client has but I would argue the potential for the struggle that the client is experiencing exists in me as well as in all human beings. I may have grown in one area of my life that allows me to function, but that doesn't hide the reality that other parts of my life are in chaos—as is true for every human being. No one has it together; we are all striving to get healed somewhere, somehow.

To illustrate my point, I will first explore and reframe two passages from the New Testament that communicate negative messages to some people. Next, I will touch upon an eloquent message on human frailty by Thomas Merton.

Reframing Negative Connotations from the Bible

Sometimes the words in biblical passages are misunderstood; readers unfamiliar with the passages draw back from the content because of strong associations with some of the texts which are based on negative experiences from the readers' past.

Consequently, consider the following passages apart from a religious context and connect them instead to this discussion on our universally shared vulnerabilities as human beings.

The first passage is found in the book of Romans, Chapter 3, verses 22b and 23a. The passage is translated as follows in the New International Version (NIV) of the New Testament: "There is no difference, for all have sinned and fall short of the glory of God."

The word *sin* is one of those emotionally charged words that usually rubs abrasively because it has been frequently overused or misued by self-righteous persons who imagine themselves as the Bible police. So, let's use a word other than *sin.* Let's go back to the Greek origin of the term and substitute that into the excerpt.

Sin is translated from the Greek verb *hamartano*, which can be translated as "missing the mark" (Arndt and Gingrich, 1979, p. 42). Let's reread the passage now: "All have missed the mark and have come short of the glory of God."

I am going to do some more work on the passage to bring it even closer to the context of our discussion. This will require some paraphrasing, which will take the reading out of the biblical context and put it into the caregiving arena.

Self-Actualization As the Glory of God

Think of the "glory of God" as Maslow's concept of a fully actualized human being who has reached a point of serenity and acceptance with whom he or she is and is functioning in life with ever-increasing joy, productiveness, and communion with others. This idea is not that far away from the biblical concept of the glory of God. Here is what Maslow (1971) says:

> First, self-actualization means experiencing fully, vividly, self-lessly, with full concentration and total absorption. It means experiencing without the self-consciousness of the adolescent. At this moment of experiencing, the person is wholly and fully human. This is a self-actualizing moment. This is a moment when the self is actualizing itself. As individuals, we all express such moments occasionally. (p. 45)

Let's use Maslow's model to identify "the glory of God" as the state when human beings become "the best they can become" and substitute this idea into the excerpt from Romans. The passage now reads this way: "All of us have missed the mark—somewhere, some-time—and have failed to become all we were meant to become as human beings."

Is this not true? Don't we all, as members of the human family, have some regrets? We have missed becoming perfect. Loose ends exist in all of our lives, and some of the dark corners of our lives are too scary to venture into. This reality puts us on a level playing field with our patients or clients. We share a common humanity of vulnera-bility, and it is only right that we do not hide this from those we help. They have a right to know, and our disclosure will give them freedom to grow.

Forgiveness and Acceptance: The Story of the Woman Caught in Adultery

The second illustration from the New Testament comes from John, Chapter 8. The story here involves some Pharisees (the morality po-lice of the time) who brought a woman to Jesus Christ and made her stand before him and a large crowd of people to endure the humilia-tion of the charge to be made against her. The Pharisees stated the woman was caught by them in the very act of adultery and, although no videotape existed in those times, the statement of those powerful men was enough to bring the charge.

The Pharisees threw the woman into the presence of Jesus because they hated Jesus and what he taught, especially that the love, grace, and forgiveness of God are greater than the commandments. The Pharisees pressured Jesus and asked him, "What are you going to do? We caught this woman red-handed. The law says she must be stoned. We are waiting for your answer."

Jesus stooped down in the dirt and started writing something. The Pharisees kept pestering him. Finally, Jesus stood up, looked the accusers in the eye and said (my paraphrase), "If any one of you has not missed the mark and can say you are cleaner than this woman, and you don't have any dark corners in your life, then you pick up a stone and kill this woman" (see John 8:7).

When this challenge was thrown down, the accusers left one by one. Afterward, Jesus was left alone with the woman. Jesus spoke to her:

> "Woman, where are they? Has no one condemned you?"
> "No one, sir," she said.
> "Then neither do I condemn you," Jesus declared. "Go now and leave your life of sin." (John 8:10-11, NIV)

The main point of this story is to illustrate that no human being can claim moral superiority over another. We have all done something wrong somewhere at some time which should hinder any inclination we might have to marginalize or condemn another person. Nonetheless, such condemnation surfaces in very subtle ways when we as caregivers work with clients.

If a caregiver places professional distance between himself or herself and the client, a hierarchy has been established and, in a very subtle way, the object of help becomes the one with the defect—or, if you please, the client metaphorically becomes the woman caught in the act of adultery. Concurrently, the caregiver becomes the Pharisee who is the dispenser of judgment—be it a pill, a form to fill out, or a program to enroll in. How unfair this is to the one who came for help.

The Universality of Human Frailty

The third illustration that makes the point that our frail, human condition is universal is eloquently disclosed by Thomas Merton.

Merton (1948), in his book *The Seven Storey Mountain,* told the story of his brother's death in an English bombing mission over Mannheim, Germany, on April 17, 1943. Merton was distressed about the war and the evils of Adolf Hitler, but, more important, Merton argued that he and the rest of the world shared responsibility for creating a time and a place where Hitler could flourish. For Merton, the sins of omission and commission perpetrated by all humanity brought on the sorrows of those dark years.

> Now it seemed that at last there really would be war in earnest. . . . It was a danger that had added to it, an almost incalculable element of dishonor and insult and degradation and shame. And the world faced not only destruction, but destruction with the greatest possible defilement: defilement of that which is most perfect in man, his reason and his will, his immortal soul.
> All this was obscure to most people, and made itself felt only in a mixture of disgust, hopelessness and dread. They did not realize that the world had now become a picture of what the majority of its individuals had made of their own souls. We had given our minds and wills up to be raped and defiled by sin, by hell itself. . . .
> There was something else in my own mind—the recognition: "I myself am responsible for this. My sins have done this. Hitler is not the only one who has started this war: I have my share in it too. . . ." (Merton, 1948, p. 248)

What stood out when I first read this passage some years ago was the idea of the Hitler in me. When Merton said his sins were as much responsible for the war as Hitler's rampages, I understood that the darkness and the evil that was in Adolf Hitler is in me too. Carl Jung (1936) alluded to this when he disucssed the "collective unconscious" which has been pictured as a circle of inner darkness in every human. This "collective unconscious" is a partial counterpart to Freud's Id as interpreted by Jung (Sharf, 1999).

Former President Bill Clinton, in an August 2000 meeting with evangelical ministers (aired on C-SPAN), stated that the Genome Project confirmed that the genetic makeup of all human beings, regardless of race or ethnicity, is 99 percent the same across the board. I contend it is the same for the whole of humanity: our total bio-psychosocial-spiritual composition as human beings is essentially the same. This is the rationale for placing ourselves at a face-to-face level with those we as caregivers have been commissioned to serve: we drink from the same fountain of life and we came forth from the same ocean of waters; we are one with our clients and patients in origin, body, mind, spirit, and susceptibility.

The Problem of Professional Distance

Knox et al. (1997) acknowledge that the use of therapist or caregiver self-disclosure is controversial. Knox and colleages state that controversy comes from the tension created by traditions of psychodynamic therapy which follows (according to some practitioners) the practices of Freud (p. 275).

The issue over nondisclosure by the therapist centers on the matter of transference. Sharf (1999) stated that transference in Freudian psychoanalysis was the patient's emotional response to the therapist. According to Sharf, Freud believed that patients would transfer repressed feelings about family members and redirect them onto the relationship with the therapist. Consequently, the role of the therapist should be as unobtrusive as possible so that this transference can be fully expressed. Hence, the patient would recline on a couch and the therapist would sit out of sight of the patient (Sharf, 1999, pp. 9-10).

Despite the persistent paradigm of the distant therapist, which may be either an understanding or misunderstanding of Freud (Wachtel, 1993, p. 208)—and which is vociferously insisted upon by some members of the psychotherapy elite—a group of helpers, myself included, embraces the sharing of self as a means of building an authentic, open relationship with a client. Knox et al. (1997) describe those therapists who advocate self-disclosure:

> Those with humanistic, existential, and eclectic orientations, on the other hand, claim to use this intervention more freely, equating realness with a fully open, honest, genuine, and personally involved stance (Simon, 1988) and viewing therapist self-disclosure as a means of demystifying the psychotherapy process (Kaslow et al., 1979). (p. 274)

Knox and colleagues (1997) conducted a qualitative analysis of the effects of therapist self-disclosure and concluded that helpful self-disclosures "(a) occurred when these clients were discussing important personal issues, (b) were perceived as being intended by therapists to normalize or reassure clients, and (c) consisted of a disclosure of personal non-immediate information about the therapists"

(p. 274). Though some clients in this analysis expressed negative feelings indicating that self-disclosure violated therapist-client boundaries, the overall results of self-disclosure as chosen by the therapists in the study was positive.

Hazards of Self-Disclosure

It is appropriate at this point to clarify some of the parameters of self-disclosure that are in keeping with the context of my story. One belief I have expressed is that the therapist who has experienced suffering parallel to the suffering of his or her client has a deeper understanding and greater compassion for the plight of the client. Hence, the "wounded healer" has more power to heal. Given this assumption, self-disclosure is extremely important and provides new insights for the client to help him or her cope with circumstances and see things from a new point of view (Knox et al., 1997).

Given all the above, situations occur in which self-disclosure is not appropriate. Consequently, the therapist must make the decision as to when and what he or she will disclose. Not every self-disclosure is efficacious. Concurrently, the purpose of self-disclosure is not intended for the catharsis of the therapist; it is for the benefit of the client, which then creates the benchmark for what will be disclosed (Twemlow, 1997, p. 10).

Following is an account of a personal experience I had when I was a student intern for an MSW program in which I discovered the hard way that self-disclosure and even a Rogerian approach to helping were not the best choices for every client.

I was working as a counselor for a government agency that provided services to persons with alcohol and other drug addictions. A client with whom I met had serious alcohol and substance abuse problems. Despite these addictions, he presented as a repentant individual, stating that he wanted to get his life together. In my naivete, I took the client at face value and gave to him my full empathetic attention. I offered encouragement that, indeed, he could win over his battle with drugs and alcohol. As the therapist, I did not share the same problems of substance abuse with the client, so no self-disclosure occurred in that regard. However, we did share a similar faith, so that became a point of connection and mutuality with the client. Nonetheless, I made a big mistake opening up as I did with this person. I didn't realize at the time that this individual needed a cop or a drill sergeant as a counselor rather than a facilitator who offers a warm teddy bear of affirmation.

At 2:00 a.m. following an appointment the previous day with this individual, I received a phone call at my home from this client. Since I was also a local minister at the time that I was doing social work training, my phone number was on public record. This meek and mild Dr. Jekyll had turned into an ugly Mr. Hyde: when he called at 2:00 a.m., he was roaring drunk and his rationale had ceased when the alcohol kicked in. The client admitted to blackouts and stated he did not remember making phone calls to me. For days I received calls from this client four and five times a night in the early morning hours when he was most under the influence. I had to disconnect my phone and file a complaint with the local sheriff. Yes, that warm, engaging approach became a season in hell for me.

The point of the forgone story is simply this: Be streetwise. Know your client. What you share of yourself is very case specific. You learn that a raging drunk needs a drill sergeant, but at the same time you discover that empathetic mutuality will work with another person who is suffering from stress and anxiety. In summary, an expansion of the aphorism "Know thyself" applies fittingly to the story I just told: "Know thyself; know thy client; listen to thy instincts." This is a sensible guideline for making decisions regarding both self-disclosure and a therapeutic approach.

The Therapist's Knowledge of Self and Awareness of Human Vulnerability

I have given a rationale for mutuality and transparency in a therapist-client relationship, and hopefully I have addressed some of the objections. Before we enter the next section of our exploration, it would be important to consider whether the therapist can approach a client with mutuality and transparency. If that therapist would be aware that just because he or she cannot state this mutuality for the sake of the client's best care, at least that therapist should know within himself or herself that vulnerability and humanity are shared with the client. Although it may be necessary to create distance for the sake of effective therapy in a client-specific circumstance, the therapist who functions most effectively understands that no distance exists in the common humanity between him or her and the client. Wachtel (1993) puts it this way:

> Doing psychotherapy, by its very nature, entangles the therapist in the conflicts of another human being. Short of maintaining a degree of distance I have argued throughout this book is unproductive, there is no way the therapist can entirely escape from the trials this introduces. The consequences of this enmeshment in the patient's conflicts are not entirely negative, however. If the therapist can skillfully maintain the proper balance of engagement and reflection, such immersion in the patient's interpersonal world can be a primary medium for understanding the patient's experience and the source of his difficulties. (p. 229)

Wachtel (1993) notes that the therapist not only becomes entangled, necessarily, in the affairs of the patient, but "therapists have conflicts too" (p. 233). The outcome of this admitted humanity produces these results: "In disclosing an aspect of a therapist's humanity as part of an effort to help the patient re-appropriate the full experience of her own, this comment illustrates well the issues with which this chapter has been concerned" (Wachtel, 1993, p. 234).

THE DARK SIDE OF THE CAREGIVING PROFESSIONAL'S WORLD

Regardless of the field one chooses, be it medicine, social work, psychology, or ministry, the emphasis of this writing has been that caregivers are as susceptible to the foibles of being human as those they serve.

In the opening of his chapter on countertransference, Kahn (1991) clarifies that the vulnerability of the therapist is no different than the vulnerability of the client. To illustrate this point, Kahn describes an encounter with a client that made him feel both hurt and angry.

Definition of Countertransference

Countertransference constitutes the sum of feelings and attitudes experienced by the therapist that could best be described as a reaction to the interaction the therapist has with the client. The feelings and attitudes that make up countertransference can be positive, negative, or both. Such feelings and attitudes fall into three categories:

1. "realistic responses" (i.e., the client is a friendly, attractive person),
2. "responses to transference" (i.e., the client expresses anger and the therapist feels threatened), and
3. "responses to material troubling to the therapist" (i.e., the therapist is going through a divorce, and the therapist feels envy if the client describes a happy marriage). (Kahn, 1991, pp. 118-119)

The Vulnerable Therapist

Consequently, the reality of countertransference underscores the vulnerability of the therapist or caregiver, and this vulnerability is part of the matrix in the relationship with the patient or client. Kahn retells an incident in which a client blasted him for his insensitivity. The client stated, "On Rogers' eight-point empathy scale I'd give you about a *three*" (p. 115). Note Kahn's reaction to this insult: deep down, the hurt was still struggling to make itself known.

> "I'm the one supposed to be watching the store around here," I said to myself. My defenses won the struggle, the hurt was successfully suppressed, and with relief I re-established my faith in the myth of psychotherapy: *In this room there is one distressed person with problems and one professional who has it all together.*
>
> If you were to ask me if I believe that, that I have it all together, I would honestly assure you that I believe no such thing; I know only too well how untrue that is. (p. 115)

Fortunately, Kahn was willing to share his humanity to emphasize that caregivers do not experience life as perfect people without feelings, be they good or bad. Kahn further points out that he was a client before he became a therapist. Hence, Kahn as a caregiver has a connection to those he serves because he has been in their position as well.

Nevertheless, those caregivers who are dishonest and deny their humanity open themselves to a caldron of dark behaviors that ultimately do damage to the client. Following are a few examples of a dark side in the world of caregiving professionals who are dishonest with themselves and others and fail to address their own human vulnerabilities.

PATHOLOGIES IN THE THERAPIST-CLIENT RELATIONSHIP

Issues of Power and Control

Kahn (1991) acknowledges that early analysts in the Freudian tradition wrestled with the tension that was created with the "blank screen" approach to therapy. Though the purpose was to cause the patient to disclose inner feelings as a result of the "unapproachability" of the therapist to patient interaction, some sensitive analysts realized that remaining unresponsive could be perceived by the patient as "sadistic dominance" (pp. 7-8).

Parallel to this perception of sadistic dominance in Freudian psychoanalysis, Twemlow (1997) recognizes that sadistic dominance can be a real hazard in which the therapist exploits the client in destructive ways. Twemlow asserts that such abuse of power is dangerous to the client. Twemlow (1997) has discussed several cases in which doctors have taken advantage of their authoritative positions and abused or tortured patients; some use their positions of trust to instigate sexual relations with patients, while others treat their clients in a condescending, sexist, or generally derogatory way, victimizing the very individuals they are expected to help.

Twemlow (1997) also describes a counterabuse of power in which the therapist became tormented by the patient. Twemlow stated this event was a "masochistic surrender" on the part of the caregiver: a psychiatrist overprescribed medications to a demanding and troubling patient, which resulted in a major suicide attempt by this patient. The doctor claimed he was helpless to do anything else. Twemlow argues that this masochism is an acting out of the therapist's growing hatred toward the patient (p. 8).

As documented in these stories, the potential for the therapist to be a victimizer and for the patient to become a victim is real, especially if the therapist is dishonest or has not addressed his or her own vulnerabilities.

Professionalism As a Disguise: A Place to Hide Out from Life and from Self

Some years ago I remember a discussion in one of the master of social work seminars in which I participated that explored the dark side of why some enter fields of social work and psychology. Facilitators at that workshop acknowledged that a de facto understanding exists within various branches of the helping professions that acknowledges many persons enter these fields because of their own issues—and entering these professions is a good way of putting off dealing with your own problems.

Kahn (1991) cites Carl Rogers regarding this matter of hiding behind a professional disguise to avoid facing one's own internal issues:

> Therapists must be *genuine* or as Rogers sometimes said, "congruent." That means they must have on-going access to their own internal process, their own feelings, their own attitudes, their own moods. Rogers believed that therapists who were not receptive to the awareness of their own flow of feeling and thought would be unlikely to help clients become aware of theirs. Undoubtedly there are therapists who choose this profession because they imagine that focusing on the client's internal process is a good way of avoiding the pain and anxiety of looking at their own. Rogers teaches that this is a recipe for disaster. Becoming a therapist means taking on the awesome responsibility for facing oneself. (pp. 38-39)

I have met my share of caregiving professionals who have hidden behind their respective badges of professional authority, pulled rank, and protected themselves from scrutiny to avoid being authentic and facing their own issues of human weakness and recovery. As Kahn and Rogers aptly illustrate, hiding out in a caregiving profession to avoid facing self and one's place in a community is destructive to clients and "a recipe for disaster."

Manipulation: Use and Abuse of Clients for Self-Serving Ends

I remember a vivid experience I had with client manipulation and exploitation when I was too young and inexperienced to know fully what was happening. The era was the 1960s, and I had applied for a teaching position with the Los Angeles City Schools. I was about twenty-five years old. The position I was applying for ended up being in the cauldron of the civil rights movement among African Americans in South Central Los Angeles in 1968. Martin Luther King Jr. had been assassinated in the spring of 1968. Consequently, hostilities toward whites were at their peak at this time. To be accepted for the position I sought, I had to get medical clearance from the administration of the Los Angeles City Schools.

Complicating the clearance process was my classification of 1-Y with the Selective Service Board of the U.S. government. This was at the height of the Vietnam War; the previous year I had been called by the Selective Service or Draft Board for induction into military service. During the interview process, I indicated that I was interested in serving in the Navy, but I did not think I could handle submarine duty because of anxiety about being in enclosed places. This sparked a red flag with the Draft Board and I was sent to a psychiatrist who subsequently gave me a 1-Y classification, which I guess was like having mental "flat feet."

As an aside to my expressed fears, I probably was not too far afield in expressing these fears. At the time that I wrote this chapter, the news of the death of 113 Russian sailors in a submarine that became disabled in 325 feet of water was on the front pages (Newman et al., 2000). I cannot think of a more horrible way to die than being trapped underwater in a submarine.

Nevertheless, when I applied for this teaching position, the 1-Y classification was an albatross around my neck. I had to get clearance from a psychiatrist to be accepted for employment.

I went to see a psychiatrist whom I won't identify. When I told the doctor I needed a psychological evaluation to get clearance to teach with the Los Angeles City Schools, he refused to provide an immediate assessment. Instead, he told me that I would have to pay a large sum of money to attend one of his groups over an extended period of time as a prerequisite for an evaluation.

Despite my naivete and the pressure from this doctor, I realized I was being exploited and sought another physician who ultimately cleared me for employment.

As an aside to this experience, I was one of the few white teachers who survived the turbulent years of civil rights unrest in South Central Los Angeles. I taught seven years and endured mass school walkouts, an assault attempt by a crowd of 200 students, and an attack by a militant blackpower group that left me with mementos such as a bloody shirt and a trip to the emergency room with my bottom teeth pushed through my lower lip.

Despite these tribulations, I established some deep bonds with my students in South Central Los Angeles, and I fostered some friendships that have left with me deep impressions of affection and high regard for many of these courageous young people. I consider those years in the late 1960s and early 1970s to be some of the best I experienced as a teacher.

Concurrent to the experience I just described, Twemlow (1997) identifies hatred and envy as subconscious reasons a therapist would choose to exploit a client. The playing field is not level; the prospective client runs considerable risk if he or she is placed in a therapeutic relationship in which the caregiver has not addressed nor received help for his or her own issues.

Twemlow told the story of a therapist who expressed hatred toward a female client when he was frustrated by her failure to progress in the way he wanted her to. This woman awoke from a hypnosis session to find her therapist "touching her genitalia." When she asked the therapist what he was doing, he replied, "You have guided me to be possessed by what possessed your father." To which the patient screamed, "But my father did what he did because he hated me" (p. 9).

Issues of Dominance

Another hazard that Twemlow states can corrupt the relationship between the client and therapist is the dialectical dynamics of dominance and submission. If the therapist has not come to terms with his or her vulnerability to need to feel power over the client, problems of dominating the client can surface.

Twemlow asserts that dominance and submission are chief themes in therapist and patient relationships. He goes on to say that the professional is usually put into a role in which he or she does something to the patient. When the "something done" to the patient is combined with the therapist's "fiduciary responsibility and greater skill and knowledge," this combination becomes "a potential crucible for a pathological victim and victimizer relationship." Twemlow argues further that the relationship of exploitation perpetrated by the therapist is more than just an *iatrogenic* or clinician-caused disease. A more accurate term coined by Twemlow and a colleague is *"syndyadogenic"* (Twemlow and Gabbard, 1981). *Syndyadogenic* disease is an illness caused by the collusion of two people working together: the therapist and the patient (Twemlow, 1997, p. 9).

The Client As Guinea Pig or Curiosity

The immediate thing that comes to mind when I consider this hazard in the client-therapist relationship is related to the mistreatment of Native Americans by anthropologists in the early twentieth century. Jansen (2000), in an AP news release, wrote of the return of the brain of Ishi to members of his nation in Northern California. Ishi, a Yahi Native American who was the subject of an anthropological treatise by Alfred L. Kroeber (Heizer and Kroeber, 1979) at the University of California, suffered the indignation of having his body dissected and his brain sent to the Smithsonian Institute as a sort of scientific curiosity. It has taken the current generation of Native Americans protesting this callous dehumanizing objectification of not only a person but a race of people to initiate changes that give respect to members of indigenous cultures by the scientific community.

Despite these ethical advances in the anthropological and scientific communities, clients of therapists are often exploited as objects of study for reasons that meet a perverse need of the therapist rather than promoting progress in the field of mental health.

Twemlow (1997) refers to Stoller (1974) whom Twemlow says clarifies what it means to dehumanize the patient or client as a object. Stoller says that the fetishing of a patient occurs when the patient is engaged in a relationship as a part-object rather than a whole object— that is, "a complete human being capable of a full range of interactions as would occur in a mature relationship." The problem for the errant therapist is that relating to a person as a whole is too threatening for such a therapist. The patient who is fetished, and not seen as a whole person, becomes a more managable "bag of pathologies" in need of the special care of the therapist (p. 7).

The Client As a Drug to Meet the Therapist's Needs

This concluding problem on dysfunctional relationships between the caregiver and the client was not specifically discussed in the literature I researched. Nonetheless, when we examine this problem, it will become evident that the problem of self-medicating via the caregiving encounter is a composite of all the elements of exploitation we have just explored.

Life stressors are common experiences for all of us. Frequently, when life seems to be out of control, I have heard many persons say, "Thank God for my work. I can throw myself into my work, and this keeps me from going crazy." There is a danger connected to throwing yourself into your career to avoid dealing with personal issues. If your career is a safe, stable enterprise, it can become an intoxicating escape in which you fail to address and resolve serious problems that stand in the way of personal growth, recovery, and healing.

Without question, gaining satisfaction and solace from a career—particularly the career of caregiving—is not wrong in itself. Whatever vocation we choose, a given prerequisite for most of us is that we enjoy the work and gain satisfaction from the use of our talents. I am not saying that finding refuge in our jobs is wrong. What is wrong for the caregiver becomes a matter of degree. If one's professional role is a means to escape the unaddressed failures of one's life, the profession then becomes a drug no different from the self-medication of alcohol and street drugs to alleviate psychic pain.

M. Scott Peck (1991) described the life of Heather Barsten, a fictional character in his novel *A Bed by the Window.* Heather was a charge nurse at the Willow Glen Nursing Home. One could not find a more efficient caregiver than Heather. Willow Glen could not be the same without the passionate and dedicated labors of Heather.

Nonetheless, Heather's life was a mess. Beyond the arena of the nursing home and the locale of Heather's flawless efficiency was her personal life, which was in shambles. Heather stumbled from one abusive relationship to the next with men who mistreated her. Despite her psychiatrist's efforts to redirect the negative emotional recordings that played in Heather's mind, she was not willing to address her problems and change. Heather was not only hiding out from her troubles, she was also abusing her job at Willow Glen by using her work as her drug of choice so that she would not have to deal with issues in her life which called for change. One of the nursing home residents, Mrs. Grochowski, exposed to Heather the very fact that she was in a dead-end job because it was safe and allowed Heather to persistently avoid dealing with serious life issues:

> "Well I suppose you [Heather] might want to ask yourself what you are doing here, taking care of us old bodies. Is that what really interests you? You're so bright you could go to college. Are you going to spend your life working in a nursing home? You could do so much more."
>
> "I can't go to college. My parents are poor. You know my father drinks everything away."
>
> "There are scholarships, you know," Mrs. Grochowski countered. "You don't have to let anyone walk all over you, including your father. But I don't want to argue with you, Heather. Still, the fact is that you're maybe in a dead-end job here. You might want to ask yourself why. Do you take such good care of us because you really enjoy it—because that's all you want—or are you doing it for some other reason?"
>
> Heather could feel the stubbornness rising up from the bottom of her spine into her chest. "Why are you beating up on me, Mrs. G?"
>
> "I'm not. But if you really want to see it that way, I feel like answering it in the way I did when I was a little girl: you started it. You did ask for it, you know." (Peck, 1991, p. 80)

The point of this illustration is that Heather as a caregiver, despite her efficiency, was not in the best place either for herself or for the persons for whom she cared. Though no real exploitation occurred, Heather could be described as using her job as a form of life-avoidance medication. This is a no-win situation for both the caregiver and the patient.

This brief investigation concerned the possible hazards that can damage the relationship between a caregiver who has not come to terms with his or her humanity and the persons being served. We will now consider a fresh model of the caregiver/patient relationship based on the oneness of human experience.

A NEW MODEL OF THE CAREGIVER-CLIENT RELATIONSHIP

When I prepared the outline for this chapter, the pathologies I put together that affected the caregiver-client relationship were generated by personal experiences and hunches. When I did the research, I was amazed to discover that the problems were more than hunches; they were documented encounters between caregivers and clients in diverse settings. The ubiquity of the pathological problems in caregiver-client relationships (even though such problems represent a small percentage of client-caregiver interactions taken as a whole) makes the case for the theme in this book: that the caregiver's common humanity and susceptibility to err, exploit, and hurt the client can be greatly reduced if such a caregiver exercises his or her craft with a full acceptance of his or her humanness and concurrent fallibility and weakness. This acceptance of weakness on the part of a caregiver is the pathway to strength and effectiveness in a therapeutic relationship.

Biblical Benchmarks

Two pieces of wisdom are found in the New Testament that provide guidelines for restructuring of the relationship between the caregiver and the person he or she serves. The first is the mutual confession of faults; the second is the power attained through experiencing weakness. These two principles, though certainly not new, constitute my proposal for a fresh model of the caregiver-patient relationship.

Mutual Confession, Mutual Acceptance

James 5:16 is the first of these two pieces of wisdom. The passage reads, "Confess your sins to each other and pray for each other so that you may be healed" (NIV).

The context of this passage relates to a church setting and the promotion of harmony among members of a congregation in a first-century setting. This concept of mutual confession removes barriers between us and our fellow human beings according to commentary by Barclay (1976a, p. 131). Barclay cautions that the verse does not imply that we should blurt out everything without discrimination, because some kinds of confession can do more harm than good, depending on the audience. Consequently, a way to rephrase James 5:16 based on the thesis of this book would be: "Do not be afraid to confess and acknowledge your humanity with one another, so in fact the process of therapy can proceed without barriers." A caveat to this principle is this: If the caregiver realizes that it would be counterproductive to disclose something to his or her client, at least that therapist has an understanding about himself or herself that puts the therapist on the same human ground as the client, not above the client.

The Story of the Good Samaritan

This brings to mind another story in the New Testament about authenticity that was told in Luke 10:25-37. The story is known as the "Parable of the Good Samaritan." In this parable told by Jesus Christ, a man who was traveling was accosted by robbers, beaten up, and left for dead. Two religious dignitaries came by after the vicious crime occurred and refused to stop and help the man. However, a Samaritan came upon the injured man soon after the "pious ones" left him for dead, and this Samaritan went down into the ditch, nursed this man's wounds, and financed his food and lodging so the man could recover and continue on his way.

The point in the parable for us as caregivers comes with the understanding the Samaritan had about himself. During the time of this story, Samaritans were racial outcasts in the culture of which they were a part. The bigwigs, (i.e., the priests and the lawyers) had an image to protect. Stopping to help a dirty, beaten victim of a robbery was not going to help the lofty ones (unless eyewitness news was there to televise their philanthropy). However, the Samaritan's situation was different: he had no reputation to defend and, as is apparent in the parable, this Samaritan was willing to enter a ditch to give merciful care to a fellow human being.

All Human Beings Walk the Same Road of Life
Between Birth and Death

This is the foundation of effective care: As fellow members of the human species, we walk the same road of life between birth and death. Those boundaries of birth and death make us equal. I come to care for you—just as I am, failures and all—to help you get back on your feet so that you may experience healing and recovery. Hopefully, your life and my life will have become much better simply because we met along the way.

Human Imperfection Is Universal

Scott Peck has provided inspiration for many ideas presented here, and he is a model for appropriate disclosure and the removal of barriers when he reflects on his humanity as a psychiatrist.

Peck wrote *In Search of Stones* (1995), which chronicles his journey to the megaliths of England, Wales and Scotland (Stonehenge is one example)—monuments likely erected by civilizations in that part of the world during the Paleolithic and Neolithic periods. The chronicle was more than a discussion of stone formations; Peck wove a confessional into the journey as images and events caused him to reflect upon his own life. Peck was forthright about problems with addiction, infidelity in his marriage, and the problems he had building a good relationship with his children. The author's candidness hurt no one, but for me, as a fan of his writing, my respect and connection to him as a human being grew tenfold. Here is a man who is a psychiatrist and the author of numerous best-selling books. Nonetheless, he is a human being, just like I am, who is struggling with life. I experienced camaraderie with Scott Peck. When I read his confessions, I had these thoughts: "Hey! He is just like me. We put our pants on the same way. We are walking along similar paths, and his training and renown don't make him a loftier person."

In addition, I remember the gratitude and relief I felt when I read Peck's story and reconsidered the shame I felt about my own failures. I reflected this way: "Even the greatest among us are imperfect. It's okay to have shortcomings and to struggle toward healing and recovery."

The Power of Weakness

The apostle Paul is the one who communicated this wisdom to us, and he suggests an ironic dichotomy: strength comes out of weakness. Paul speaks about the power he receives from Christ: "That is why, for Christ's sake, I delight in weaknesses, in insults, in hardships, in persecutions, in difficulties. For when I am weak, then I am strong" (2 Corinthians 12:10, NIV).

The Greek word from which the translation *weak* comes is *astheneo,* which means "to be without strength" (Young, p. 1040). How is it that one can be without strength and at the same time possess great power? The answer comes from what kind of power we mean. Consider the experience my wife had when I was going through the ordeal of the panic attacks. This is what she said:

> You know, Dan, there was a special gentleness about you when you were in the midst of that terrible experience. I would not wish that ever again upon you, but I will tell you that I liked the softness and compassion it created. It was the first time you accepted your weakness and humanity without fighting it—which you could not stand in anyone else.

This is the power that weakness creates. From the context of the New Testament, it is a power of God that cannot be released unless a person such as Paul or myself has reached the end of all resources. Barclay (1976b) stated, "for always man's extremity is God's opportunity" (p. 260). This presupposes that even if Christianity is not a person's faith a power exists beyond us that cannot be accessed unless we come to the very end of our complacent selves.

REFLECTION

In this new approach I am proposing, we look at caregiving beyond the reaches of human capacity. In my case, since my frame of reference is the Christian faith, the power of God enters the picture when we reach the end of our strength and abilities to help those in the professions we have been called to serve. So just what is this new approach to the caregiver-patient relationship? We have discussed its details; here are its main concepts in a nutshell.

Common Humanity

Admit and embrace the humanity that the caregiver shares with the patient. In our hearts, we don't place ourselves above the person, even though the clinical setting may not make it appropriate to share such information with the client. At least we know and demonstrate to the client by our actions and genuine compassion that we accept the client as a fellow human being with dignity.

Weaknesses Are Assets

The irony of our roles as caregivers is that our very weaknesses, which we think would stand in the way of serving our clients, may be our greatest assets.

Concurrent with this ironic connection of our personal weakness to ultimate therapeutic power, I would propose that a fresh approach to the caregiving model would be to pair clients with therapists who have been down similar roads. For example, I have a deep understanding of what it means to suffer a panic attack and remember what it was like to have a ruminating brain that was out of my control. I know what it is to reach out for help. I know what the pain feels like, and I know what the recovery (which is ongoing) feels like as well. I know what the trademarks of panic feel like, and my empathy for a client with the same experience is deeper because I have been there.

This is not to say that a caregiver has to experience everything his or her client experiences to be an effective helper. Nevertheless, the most effective help, I think, comes from the wounded healer. The bond with the client who exclaims, "You mean you have had this experience, too?" runs deep, and the healer's statement, "I understand," is far more than empty words.

Chapter 9

Toward a Fresh Model of the Caregiver-Client Relationship: The Oneness of Human Experience—Part 2

Emil Authelet

INTRODUCTION

The Therapeutic Evaluation of the Therapist

Part of every training program at the heart of the caregiving process is the therapeutic evaluation of the therapist. The psychiatrist training to become an analyst goes through analysis so that he or she can work out of an inner level of wholeness in treating others. The clinical psychologist, social worker, psychiatric technician, marriage and family therapist, or pastoral counselor have all undergone some form of psychological examination for the same purpose. Underlying this is the need for the caregiver to deal with his or her own issues before entering into a therapeutic relationship with a client. Beneath this is the reality that to help another, one's own issues must not interfere with the healing process but instead enhance it.

Dishonest Therapists in Hiding

No failsafe system is in place to safeguard this practice as intended. Too many horror stories are told of persons entering this field hoping subconsciously to figure themselves out. Others may be on power trips and see this as a way of manipulating others for their own needs. Consider the psychiatrist on a psych ward at a state mental institution who is as ill as many of his patients but who believes as long as he is working there he cannot be as ill as those who are patients under his care. Likewise, think of the pastoral counselor who is in reality a predator and hides within his profession looking for vulnerable people to victimize. In addition, envision the caregiver who is seeking to work out who she is at the expense of the clients she is supposed to be helping.

One characteristic to be found in each of the pathologies just described is that of professional distance. These individuals cannot tolerate exposure for the truth will reveal them. Consequently, these persons develop ways of hiding. Correspondingly, "professionalism" in and of itself is a potential way of hiding ("I'm the therapist; you're the patient").

Caregiving Is a Gift of Self

Caregiving is the gift of oneself within a therapeutic relationship in which the approach is between equals, not the therapist being okay and the client not okay. We can work toward ongoing healing and wholeness. Good therapy and healing takes place among equals.

Within the therapeutic relationship of caregiving, there is always a level of personal vulnerability and conjoint susceptibility to the vicissitudes of the human experience which the therapist shares with the client. When this cannot take place because of the unmet needs of the therapist, the client is cheated and hurt by the process that occurs. For therapy to work an openness and vulnerability must be present on the part of the therapist that has a ring of truth which the client can come to trust.

The client must be able to know and say to himself or herself, "The therapist is not playing games with me or using me for personal ego needs." This is absolutely essential to the client's healing. The client cannot be expected to abandon falsity when the therapist has not. The purpose of a psychological game is to avoid such intimacy. The healing process is based on the potential for awareness, spontaneity, and intimacy.

The DSM-IV Is a Biography of the Therapist and the Client

All one has to do is examine the *Diagnostic and Statistical Manual of Mental Disorders,* Fourth Edition, (APA, 1994) to see a portrait of human frailty and to understand how much of it is shared in varying degrees by the majority. The DSM-IV informs us that caregiving will be a needed practice as long as humanity survives on this planet. At the same time, the DSM-IV is biographical of both therapist and client. This is what Henri Nouwen (1972) addressed in his book, *The Wounded Healer: Ministry in Contemporary Society.*

THE DARK SIDE OF CAREGIVING

Caregiving within our society has not escaped its dark side, as public reports chronicle. I worked for a mainline Protestant denomination for eleven years in the field of conflict resolution. Hardest for me in this role was handling cases of clergy sexual misconduct, cases of sexual harassment, and ministerial abuse. What is true here is also true for all areas of caregiving: abuse should never be present. It is the antithesis of the calling for ministering to health and wholeness. Those who are charged with working with life's most vulnerable persons should never be or become abusers themselves. Those who entrust themselves to our care deserve the assurance that we are present for their healing and for nothing else. In every healing relationship, the therapist always receives a life gift from the one he or she is working with. Nonetheless, this is the grace of the relationship and never the purpose.

Dominance Over a Client

Therapy can become a weapon of power and control, but where does that leave the client? The weak remain weakened further, rather than helped into independence and meaningful forms of interdependence. The vulnerable are made more vulnerable in order to serve the needs of the therapist. The broken remain broken and in the process may lose what they did have going for them. In each of the previous illustrations, the therapist may be guilty of adding the final straw to an already overwhelming emotional load and, as a result, may cause the client to "break." There are no guarantees within the therapeutic process, but one can be relatively certain of the outcome of professional abuse: this misuse of trust is devastating.

Professionalism As a Disguise

The guise of professionalism can become a place to hide from life and a place to avoid dealing with one's own issues. Accordingly, the guise of professionalism can become a means by which the client is used and often abused. Here, again, the focus is on the needs of the therapist rather than those of the client. A therapist might internally rationalize such an approach in this manner:

> "Since you are coming to me for help, I can hide behind the mask of the helper, thus keeping you distanced so you will not discover the depths of my own need." The professional jargon of the therapist and the labeling of the client, first as "client" or "patient" then as "neurotic" or "obsessive-compulsive," further establishes this disguise.

> "I'm OK—You're not OK," and I am here to remind you of that while defending and disguising my own "not okayness."

Manipulation, Use, and Abuse

Therapy can involve the manipulation, use, and abuse of clients for self-serving ends. There is always the temptation to keep clients engaged longer than they need for the sake of the therapist. It can happen very easily when income is scarce or the therapist's plans require increased income. I remember being in my dentist's chair when the dentist's wife called to tell him the transmission on her car failed. She obtained an estimate at the garage where it had been towed and told the dentist what the bill would be. Since the dentist and his wife were both friends of mine, I asked him how much it was going to cost. The dentist replied, "Two crowns and three root canals." Since I was already in the chair with my mouth open, I figured the work being done on me would be one of those procedures helping to pay for the car repair.

The point of this humorous anecdote is that care and service providers must understand their own motives and have a clear sense of professional calling to be objective in dealing with clients. Abuses can become disguised as "caring" invitations. Nonetheless, abuse by any other name is still abuse.

The Client As a Guinea Pig

New therapies, techniques, and personal discoveries may be used without proper training, expertise, or preparation. Professional competition, personal advancement, and peer rivalry can influence a clinician to experiment with a new technique or model of therapy. None of this is threatening in and of itself until it clouds discernment and takes the focus away from client needs.

A caregiver is obligated by decency and ethical responsibility to inform the client when something new is being introduced and tested in the therapy setting. Such experimentation should be done openly, with client agreement, and with the full disclosure of procedures to maintain therapist-client trust.

The Client As a Curiosity

Every caregiver has exceptional and at times interesting cases. However, if the notoriety of the client overshadows the real need of the client in the perception of the therapist, then the focus may shift, and the client is not well served. The relationship between the therapist and client is corrupted if the therapist's point of view is similar to this:

> I must keep this person engaged in therapy with me because I want to be able to claim him or her as a client and share discoveries and information with colleagues that come from the sessions I have with such a unique individual.
>
> Perhaps the needs of the client would be better served by a therapist who specializes in areas other than mine, but my needs prevent me from making the needed referral.

Clearly in this situation the client's needs are secondary to the therapist's needs, which is unacceptable.

The Client As a Drug

The client can become a clandestine drug to meet the therapist's needs. Parallel to the previous discussion, some clients present with very unusual needs or are high-profile persons who can become a bragging point among colleagues or even result in a degree of sensationalism for the therapist.

Sessions for a therapist may be very predictable and almost routine day after day when, unexpectedly, one client arrives who challenges and enlivens the process as few others might. The therapist may get hooked into the high this provides and find himself or herself tolerating the other patients while planning ahead with a degree of excitement for the "special one." In the end, the client is usually the loser.

Refusing to Refer

What happens with the client whose needs are beyond the capabilities of the therapist? Making a referral is hard for many therapists to do, as they perceive it as a sign of weakness or incompetence on their part. No therapist can serve everyone any more than one medical doctor can treat all patients. We all have our limits, personalities, abilities, diagnostic skills, and blind spots. We have our prejudices and they too can interfere with the therapeutic process. We also have our specialties—what we like working with most. Not all specialize in addictions, depression, obsessive compulsions, or multiple personalities. The best thing we can do for the healing of clients that are not best treated by us is to make an appropriate referral and to follow up on the client's progress with genuine concern for the person's wellbeing.

Creating Unnecessary Dependence

Often the client is kept dependent because of the therapist's needs. To terminate with a client prematurely due to waning interest or to postpone termination because of one's own needs are equally dysfunctional. With insurance companies becoming more involved in the terms and duration of treatment, this is less of a problem.

Nonetheless, many clients are still responsible for the payment of their own fees. Consequently, the termination of services to a private-pay client should reflect the quality of care shown throughout the healing process. The nest is no longer needed when the bird is ready to fly on its own. A sensitive therapist knows when the treatment has reached that point and negotiates the termination with the client.

Whenever the real need of the client is the main focus and the therapist is working at her or his best, the following qualities become obvious throughout the process to all involved: (1) healthy give and take, (2) healthy authenticity, and (3) a growing progress within the healing process. These qualities of a good therapeutic relationship are deeply satisfying to all concerned. This is what real caregiving should be about.

A NEW MODEL OF THE CAREGIVER-CLIENT RELATIONSHIP

Healthy Authenticity

Healthy authenticity involves connecting to the client in a way that does not blur boundaries. A healthy relationship between therapist and client is one in which both engage in relating at such a level that genuine healing can take place. Within the medical model there is always a hierarchical relating that can undermine the psychological and emotional healing of the patient. It can also hinder the therapist's ability to share oneself with the patient. This is why a new model is needed.

Skill and knowledge, coupled with a level of care and concern, are prerequisites for creating a good therapeutic relationship. Nevertheless, the connection of the therapist with the patient is more than that. The patient and therapist are two persons on equal ground. The therapist is slightly different because he or she is farther along on the road of healing and is encountering the real needs of the patient who has not yet reached such a point on the same road.

This illustration establishes a boundary and differentiation of both becoming as one, yet maintaining all the ego boundaries needed for a healthy relationship. The therapist knows who the therapist is, who the client is, and why they are in relationship. Likewise, the client knows who the therapist is, who the client is, and why they are in relationship. Beyond that, "I'm OK and You're OK." We meet as equals.

The Healthy Therapeutic Relationship

We have just explored some qualities of an authentic therapeutic relationship within the context of a healing process. In addition, one of the graces of this healing process is the experiencing of what theology calls an atonement—resulting in a reconciliation with God/others/self/life.

Atonement could be described as the process of the client coming out of brokenness and alienation with the help of a therapist. The process takes the client from and through the brokenness and alienation of the past to new levels of growth in which the client in partnership with the therapist experiences acceptance and unconditional love. This acceptance comes first from God, and then in the therapeutic relationship. Healing has taken place to the degree that the client is able to return the acceptance and unconditional love given by the therapist. In other words, healing takes place within the relating and the relationship that offers it.

God chose to relate to us because it is our deep need and because it is the need intrinsic within love itself. Love must love. Love cannot not love. Love heals. Love is always healing.

The Therapist-Client Relationship

The therapist-client relationship is that of the "wounded healer" helping another heal. One of the basic reasons traditional psychiatry and psychoanalysis have failed as much as they have is due to this missing element. The healing is in the relationship, and the medical model is not built upon such a relationship. Of course the therapist and client relate in a medical model, but interaction is impersonal and equivalent to business transactions made with other professionals, such as a dentist, an auto mechanic, or an attorney. We pay the psychiatrist for services rendered and for his or her expertise. We rarely know psychiatrists as persons, and even more rarely do we engage such clinicians in the therapeutic relationship model just described. Clinical treatment without a give-and-take relationship with the clinician does not help to lead one into awareness, spontaneity, and intimacy. Healing is revealed from the inside out. For healing to occur inside the client, the therapist must be part of that life-generating process which occurs from the inside out.

Understanding the Vulnerability Involved

Understanding the vulnerability, need, and process of the client is absolutely essential to the establishment of a healthy therapist-client relationship. For example, when I met Bonnie she was coming out of her involvement with a cult, one that had nearly cost Bonnie her life. Many of Bonnie's friends died before they could make a similar exodus from this dangerous group. When she first considered making the break, she turned to a family friend who was a caregiver. As she tried to share her story with him and ask for his help, he began making sexual advances toward her. She could not have been more vulnerable when she approached him for help; what she got in return was someone taking advantage of her vulnerability, trying to fill his own needs.

Where did this leave her? She was experiencing exploitation within the cult; then she was receiving more exploitation when she sought help. Caregiving exists for the need of the client. The profession exists for the well-being of those being served. It is absolutely essential that the caregiver understand the level of vulnerability of the client and respond appropriately to the person's real need by being spiritually, ethically, morally, and legally responsible in protecting the client, guarding the therapeutic process, and working for the healing of the client in the fullest capacity of his or her capabilities. This is the full responsibility of the therapist and anything less than this is his or her full responsibility as well.

Being There for Others

Caregiving is for the benefit of others. Caregiving is for the benefit of some very wounded others. Caregiving is an extension of the self on behalf of these others. Out of our own personal suffering and the lessons of grace learned, we share of ourselves with these others in their need and pain and love them to health and wholeness. This is how the process is ordained to work. And it does! Critical transformations do take place in many lives, and this is one of the major keys to how well it works in the therapist. When I am in need and I turn to a therapist for help, what I want most is someone who has a listening heart, an understanding mind, and a compassion strong enough to enter my pain and help me both understand it and a find a healthy, meaningful way through it. Caregiving is exhausting work. It is also life-gifting and healing. Thank God for caregivers such as this. They are indeed the salt of the earth.

Chapter 10

Reflections on John Powell's Book
Fully Human, Fully Alive:
A Dialogue Between Emil Authelet
and Daniel Langford

Introduction by Daniel Langford

On September 8, 2000, I flew to Phoenix and spent two days with Emil and his wife, Donna, at their "casita" in Sun City West, Arizona. Besides receiving "red carpet" pampering from my hosts, our purpose in meeting was to bring together the elements of our story into the integrated whole that you have so far experienced in the journey with us.

One of the highlights during these two days was dialoging together over a tape recorder. What follows is our discourse relating to the main points of Powell's book, *Fully Human, Fully Alive.*

WHAT IT MEANS TO BE SET FREE THROUGH THE RESTRUCTURING OF OUR THOUGHTS AND OUR PERCEPTIONS OF OURSELVES

DANIEL LANGFORD: When I think of John Powell, I think of being free from negative thoughts and negative perceptions of self.

I remember when I called you during the most intense periods of panic I experienced in the summer of 1999 that you instantly recommended Powell's book for therapeutic reading. Nevertheless, when I ordered his book, I had to wait a week for it to arrive. This wait was agonizing. Waiting for the book was like waiting for the BuSpar to kick in, and I was very impatient for relief, regardless of where this relief came from. Despite the agonizing wait, the book finally arrived and, as you predicted, the reading of *Fully Human, Fully Alive* was a healing experience for me.

The most important thing that I remember when you spoke to me in August of 1999 is that you said the frightened child within me needs a new vision. This is the essence of *Fully Human, Fully Alive:* vision therapy. Please comment on this.

EMIL AUTHELET: The main thing that Powell is saying is that thoughts generate feelings. And then, we act out the feelings. What happens if I am convinced in my thinking that I am a failure? Think about yourself. You say in your mind, "I have this class of troubled kids. I have really failed. My goals were not achieved." When you are thinking this way, you will perceive yourself as a failure, and that creates panic and negative emotions about yourself. Hence, one way we act out those emotions is by running. This is the fight-or-flight response. You might believe there is nothing that you can fight, so in the face of this apparent failure, you will literally, figuratively, emotionally, and spiritually run.

Now, the key to changing this scenario is not to change the feelings but to change the thoughts. The task is to reality-test and come back and discover who I really am. Restructured thought allows you to say, "Even if I fail in the classroom, I am not a failure." When you get that thought and that understanding, the feelings change. You are no longer panicked. You may be troubled by what happened in the classroom, but you can see it for what it really is. You are not involved in a failure; you are not a failure yourself.

The Perception and Consequences of Failure in the Workplace

DL: What you are talking about here is experienced in one way or another by millions of people, particularly when it comes to our careers and our perceived successes or failures in those careers. Success or failure in a career can mean the difference between a secure income or financial ruin. Plenty is at stake in a successful job performance.

Concurrently, circumstances are not always in your favor. I remember an experience in which I was trying to do my best on a job, and the boss was someone who could not be pleased. I lost that job, and at the same time, experienced a deep sense of failure over the termination. There *was* a failure that had to be dealt with, and in that experience I found it very hard to separate who I was as a person from the experience of being told I was not competent to do the job.

EA: Here, again, it is the thought that dictates the feeling and the action. So the boss says you are a failure. But are you?

Failure on a Job Is Not *Failure As a Human Being*

DL: The perception of failure comes from within the person.

EA: The sense of failure does come from within the person and that is a person's self-perception or, as transactional analysis puts it, a person's self-awareness.

There are jobs that I cannot handle. There are jobs in my scope of professional training that I may have a great deal of difficulty with. Nonetheless, if I fail in those attempts, am I a failure? The problem with the thought process is, "My identity is in that job. Therefore, if I fail on that job, then I am a failure as a person." When you or I perceive that we are failures as human beings, we are right back into the family-of-origin dynamics carrying all of that shame and guilt. The thought is, "I failed because I am a failure."

No! These are not marks of us being failures as human beings. The reasons I fail on a job may be many:

1. I may have not had the resources I needed.
2. I may have not had the expertise and skill necessary to do the job.
3. Maybe I didn't have the support from the boss I needed.
4. Maybe it was a combination of all of the above put together.

Nevertheless, *I am not a failure as a human being.*
When I maintain this way of thinking—that I am not a failure as a human being—which is reality, then I can handle failures differently that I experience on the job. I can learn from the experiences and analyze them. I can get help from others to see where I was right, where I was wrong, where I was strong, and where I was weak. I can learn from the encounter so that I will never let myself get in that position again, because I am not a failure.

I am not going to have panic attacks over a disappointing situation. I am going to feel unhappy that I failed, but I am not going to feel bad about being me. There is a major difference between how I feel about something that has happened to me versus how I feel about who I am as a person.

Manipulation and Intimidation in Contemporary Corporations and Social Institutions

EA: Our society, especially with the advent of the Industrial Revolution, is based on the pressure of making people feel they can fail and be failures so you can push such persons to the limit on the job and get the last ounce of strength out of them.

DL: This is destructive to people.

EA: Yes, this is destructive. Nevertheless, the bottom line is that instilling a fear of failure in people makes money. You can take people, put them in jobs, and beat them to death with the result that such people will blame themselves if things don't work out. Furthermore, corporate structures are built on making people feel that their identity is the job.

DL: We cannot change the way corporations do business or manipulate people, but we can change the perception of who we are.

EA: What I said about corporations also applies to the structures of churches. We do the same thing in church. We as ministers will preach to people how bad they are, and we keep such persons under pressure with this intimidating message: "You are lucky to be here. Don't go someplace else." Hence, we work on the negative emotions of people to keep them feeling bad about themselves in order to keep them hooked. This is a manipulation to keep the congregants coming back.

The Healing Power of Alcoholics Anonymous

EA: One of the greatest things that ever happened was the conception and birth of Alcoholics Anonymous. Alcoholics Anonymous started telling people the truth. The truth communicated was this: "You need help. You need God in your life. You need a higher power. You can't do it on your own."

Furthermore, Alcoholics Anonymous communicates this hope to those seeking recovery: "You are not a failure just because you have failed. You can be a winner. Work the steps. You are worth loving. Start living like a winner."

This same kind of hope needs to be communicated in church settings. The message of a church which will communicate hope would read like this: "You may have failed, but God says he loves you because you are worth loving."

A Religious Emphasis on the Negative Side of Humanness

DL: I remember in my own religious training how much emphasis was placed on the negative side of our humanness, i.e., sin, without providing a message of hope and of God's love. Is not the grand theme of biblical message found in Jesus' words in John 3:16? "For God so loved the world that he gave his one and only Son, that whoever believes in him shall not perish but have eternal life" [NIV].

EA: Yes.

DL: Consequently, the grand theme of our Christian faith is not that we are bad, unredeemable people. The message is that we are a creation worthy to be loved which means, further, that we can have the freedom to love ourselves. Nevertheless, the message that we are bad people is the message that has been emphasized in so many of our churches.

Now, if I understand what you just stated, the "You are a bad person" message is a way of manipulating and controlling people. Am I correct?

EA: Yes. Such a negative message is very often a manipulative thing. That is why some denominations flourish. People are manipulated to keep them focused in one train of thought. Anything outside that train of thought is wrong or less than what you have if you are part of the denomination. This builds institutions.

John Calvin and the Total Depravity of Man

DL: What comes to mind is the history behind the negative message that we are bad people. Didn't John Calvin [1509-1564] preach this stuff [see Weeks, 1999]?

EA: Yes. Total depravity.

DL: So what about this? Why? John Calvin is an integral part of Protestant heritage and theology.

EA: Okay. If I share with you the fact that you cannot really earn your own salvation because anything that you would attempt to do can have sinful or mixed motives, this does not communicate that you in your core being are a horrible person. However, if I communicate that you as a human being are not worth loving or worth dying for, as declared in John 3:16, then I have misconstrued the biblical message.

Christ says to each of us, "You are worth loving, but you can't make it in this life without help. So I am going to give you my salvation or rescue as a gift. Once my gift of grace becomes a part of you, I am going to help you discover the wonderful, beautiful, unrepeatable creation of God that you are."

DL: When you read the history of John Calvin's life, you discover that he was a very mean-spirited person.

EA: He was.

DL: Calvin fought with his contemporaries and sought to silence the voices of those who disagreed with him. This is the heritage that has been passed down to us today. There is stuff in the histories of our ancestors that has not been resolved.

EA: There are many good things that came from Calvin in terms of his Christology. Nevertheless, much of the communication is negative—parent stuff.

Theology in a Psychological Framework

EA: What I pointed out in Chapter 5 is that all of this comes together when you take theology out of the philosophical framework where Calvin and other reformers have placed it and put theology in a psychological framework. The key is not to focus on the doctrine of theology as much as to focus on the relationships among God, self, and others, which is what a psychological framework provides.

The psychological framework for theology is what John Powell uses. Powell's question, as I interpret his writing, is simply this: "How do you relate to God, to others, and to self?" Though our deeds may be sinful and miss the mark, we are still persons who are worthy to be loved. The summum bonum is when Christ's

Spirit makes you a loving human being toward God, others, self, and creation.

DL: John Powell and other contemporary prophets appear to be providing us with a clearer revelation of the essence of the biblical message.

EA: Using a new paradigm such as psychology instead of philosophical doctrine does not negate everything from the past. Nevertheless, we need to allow the adult in us to test what is real and applicable from past teachings to the biblical message. From my perspective, there are points in Calvin's presentation which are a manipulation of scripture, rather than what scripture is truly teaching.

DL: We are talking about challenging the authoritative paradigms of the past, such as the teachings of John Calvin on human depravity, and reconsidering the impacts of such an emphasis upon human beings today of whom so many need to know they are loved by God and have the freedom to love themselves.

Cracks in a Creedal Structure of Faith

EA: Denominations were built on creeds, and the creeds were never examined. When we reexamine the creeds and the contexts in which they were formulated, some of the structure begins to fall apart. A good example of this is what is happening to the Roman Catholic Church. The Roman Catholic Church has a strong theological position communicated by the Vatican, which says marriage is a sacrament, thus, no one is allowed to divorce. Furthermore, divorced persons are not welcome in the Catholic Church because of this theological position. Nevertheless, many parish priests in America welcome divorced persons, and this creates a tension between doctrine and practice.

Consequently, two standards exist. One is the standard taught by the church's ecclesiastical authority in the Vatican, and the other is the standard practiced by some American churches, and the two are diametrically opposed. Some American Catholic Churches simply wink at the teaching and do what they are going to do anyway, because these churches know they will not change the mind of the Vatican.

DL: The foundational teaching has not been changed, so many churches are giving only a superficial appearance of compliance with Catholic doctrine.

EA: The foundational teaching has not been changed because if you change that, you destroy the whole superstructure that you have built on top of the teaching. If marriage is a sacrament, then you cannot allow divorce. If marriage is a sacrament, then the Church controls it because the church is the dispenser of the grace. Consequently, no marriage is legal unless it is sanctioned by the Church.

DL: So people don't get married and just live together.

EA: Or they are Protestants and live in sin.

Let Life Question You

DL: I would like to explore another element of John Powell's message in *Fully Human, Fully Alive*. Powell [1976] quoted Viktor Frankl [1984] when he suggested to his readers, "let life question you," rather than the reciprocal of you questioning life [Powell, 1976, p. 71]. This means that when one analyzes a life event, one does not ask, "Why is this happening to me?" Instead, one considers, "What questions is life asking me in my response to what is happening?"

Powell illustrates these ways in which life asks questions:

> The needy, unattractive person asks me how much I can love. The death of a dear one asks me what I really believe about death and how profitably I can confront loss and loneliness. A beautiful day or a beautiful person asks me how capable I am of enjoyment. Solitude asks me if I really like myself and enjoy my own company. . . . Success and failure ask me to define my ideas of success and failure. Suffering asks me if I really believe I can grow through adversity. [p. 71]

Would you comment on this?

EA: An experience happens, and instead of saying "Why me?" my responses might be these: "What can I learn from this? What can I take from this? What can I share with others as a result of this?" The whole orientation is outward.

Now trace it back. You quoted John 3:16 earlier. God loves, so what happens? God gives. The orientation is outward. God's orientation is toward you and toward this world that He loves.

When a tragedy happens in my life, immediately my negative thinking (or the little child inside me) turns the event toward me and asks, "Why me? Why is this happening to me?"—Well, why not? Nevertheless, we ask the questions and turn them inward.

The opposite of inward questioning is an outward response. Here is how the questioning changes. As stated above, I might ask, "What can I learn here? How is this going to help me grow? What is my life going to be when I have gotten through this experience? How will I share this with others?" The whole orientation is outward because love moves outward.

When I ask the question, "Why me?" what I am really saying is that I don't deserve this. Distorted thinking would make us believe that God or life is punishing us. Outward thinking, on the other hand, would help us realize that God might be involved in our circumstances to help us in a special way. The fully alive person can have this outward "How will this benefit me?" hopefulness rather than the inward and negative "Why is this happening to me?" hopelessness.

DL: This is a good point in our discussion to consider what Powell (1976) said, "are the five essential steps into the fullness of life" (pp. 14-18). In the forgone dialogue, we have explored Step 1: *"To Accept Oneself"* (pp. 14-15). We will now jump from Step 1 to Step 3: *"To Forget Oneself in Loving"* (p. 16).

Forgetting Oneself in Loving

EA: Christ is our example in giving himself for the world. Look at many of the individuals who are in that world; here is a related story.

I grew up in a town in rural New England, and we had several lakes in that town. We always took chances in the winter and spring as kids by being out on the ice. Sometimes the ice was pretty thin.

I remember playing hockey in those days and you couldn't stand still. If you stood still, you would go through the ice because it was so thin. You had to keep moving; you could not have a goalie because he couldn't stand there and guard one spot without going through the ice.

Inevitably, we had a kid that went through the ice. The fire department was called, and this fireman, an older man, went out to rescue the child that went through. During the rescuing process, this fireman started to have chest pains while he was trying to save the kid who will drown if he doesn't get help. So, the fireman, who is having a heart attack, doesn't turn back. He keeps going. Eventually, the fireman gets the young boy and brings him back to shore. The fireman sealed his own doom by rescuing the boy because he was having a heart attack, yet took the time to complete the rescue. The fireman died shortly after the boy was brought safely to shore. Later, some said that if the fireman had quit and not persisted in the rescue of the young boy, he could have survived his heart attack.

Here is the point. The fireman knew he was having a heart attack, and he probably knew he was going to die. The fireman had an outward orientation. This outward orientation told the fireman, "That kid is going to die if I don't get there." So the fireman kept going.

What happens with most of us when a tragedy occurs is that we go within ourselves, and we become self-absorbed and self-oriented. The natural inclination is to take care of yourself first. Powell, however, states that the outward orientation is the fully human, fully alive experience.

The Healing of the Inner Child and the Outward Expression of Love

DL: Explain how Powell balances the healing of our Inner Child with the outward expression of love and concern for others.

EA: If I don't heal—if the Inner Child is not healed—I cannot help you. I can't help anybody. Until I have healed within, I am self-absorbed. I know I am healed when my orientation shifts from self to others.

DL: This is a good description of a healer: become healed and, as a result, help in healing others.

EA: How do I know that God is real in my life? I am giving myself for others.

Authenticity

DL: Let's go back to Step 2: *"To Be Oneself"* (pp. 15-16). In this step, Powell discusses the principle of authenticity and describes it as follows:

> Fully alive people are liberated by their self-acceptance to be authentic and real. Only the people who have joyfully accepted themselves can take all the risks and responsibilities of being themselves. [p. 15]

> How do you understand self-acceptance and authenticity?

EA: If I achieve self-acceptance, I can be at home with you or anyone else and not be concerned about what I must do to be sure I will be liked. If I have to change who I am to be liked by every new person, I have lost my authenticity. I don't even know who I am. I am not myself with anybody. I only become what I think another person wants me to be so that person will like me.

The authentic person says this instead: "Here I am. This is me. It is okay to be me. I am "me" with everyone I meet. If there are three people who know me and get together in the same room to talk, these persons will discover that I am the same with all three of them together as I was with them one to one.

DL: You are not a chameleon who changes color with each new situation.

EA: I become a chameleon when I am not authentic. If the situation changes and I am a chameleon, my color changes. Games players in social situations are best described as chameleons.

DL: David Riesman [with Glazer and Denney, 1961] wrote a book called *The Lonely Crowd*. He described "other-directed" individuals who are persons with antennae up trying to decide how to behave and fit in with each new social situation in order to be accepted. Riesman explains that such persons are not "inner directed"—that is, they are not individuals who respond to an internalized core of values and perception of self. Other-directed persons are preoccupied with responding to outward cues for socialization and acceptance with a loss of self-identity in the process [pp. 17-24, 159-160].

EA: Was his conclusion that the healthy person is the inner-directed person?

DL: Yes.

EA: Consequently, we are who we really are regardless of with whom we meet and socialize.

The Ability to Believe and Find Meaning in Life

DL: *"To Believe"* (p. 17), is Step 4 in Powell's model for achieving fullness of life. The fully human, fully alive person is one who has the ability to believe and to find meaning. Powell describes this quality as follows: "Having learned to transcend purely self-directed concern, fully alive people discover 'meaning' in their lives. This meaning is found in what Viktor Frankl calls 'a specific vocation or mission in life'" [p. 17].

We live in a society in which faith has been taken out of such important institutions as our public education system. In so many ways, spirituality, the ability to believe, and the search for purpose and meaning have taken a backseat in our fast-paced, modern world. Nevertheless, spirituality, the ability to believe, and the search for meaning are of primary importance to the fully human, fully alive person. Hence, such individuals have a spiritual core or center.

EA: God reveals our spiritual purposes individually, and this has a lot to do with the gifts he gives us. Our abilities determine the types of ministry we will have. We are here for a purpose.

God created us for himself. So, the first part of my purpose is to be God's person. When I am God's person, he will lay things on my heart and before me that I need to do in life, which will be centered in the personhood of others.

I don't live just to make money. I am here to make money so that I can give to the lives of other people. I can give to the homeless; I can give to the missions of my church; I can give to organizations that are really here to benefit the world in which we live. I am not here to be blessed; I am here to be a blessing.

DL: I communicate otherness to the middle school students I teach. I tell them that the reason they were born is to give back something to other human beings.

Viktor Frankl and Meaning in Life

EA: A life purpose has nothing to do with how you are born or who your parents may or may not be. How you were born just explains how you got here. The reason we exist is that God put us on this earth, and he has a purpose for each of us. Now, meaning is what sustains life, according to Viktor Frankl [1984]. This is the essence of his logotherapy. In Frankl's own personal experience, when he went through Auschwitz during World War II, he discovered that the only people who survived the horrors of the concentration camp were those who really believed they had a meaning and a purpose for living. Frankl stated that he saw people who were literally starving to death who would go through the bread line to take food back to the barracks and feed those who did not have the strength to get off their bunks to get their own food. The risk for these persons was that they were not allowed to bring food to others, and the punishment for smuggling food was death.

Frankl observed that the purpose for living for these compassionate risk takers was to sustain other people. These were the people who survived the horrors of the concentration camps. Those who died were preoccupied only with themselves.

A Place Called Home

DL: This brings us to Step 5: *"To Belong"* (pp. 17-18). Here is Powell's description of this step:

> The fifth and final component of the full life would no doubt be a "place called home," a sense of community. A community is a union of persons who "have in common," who share in mutuality their most precious possessions—themselves. [p. 17]

Emil, this has been a grand theme of your writings: this idea of community—"a place called home." We have so far discussed a problem in our current culture, which idolizes rugged individualism and appears to eschew mutual interdependence or community. As a result of this phenomena, you have observed that many persons are socially isolated. What else would you like to say about this topic?

EA: For you and I who grew up without a sense of belonging in our families of origin, this has been a deep and unfulfilled area of our lives. Concurrently, when you reflect upon your salvation experience—salvation literally means "rescue"—and your Christian experience, you understand that these experiences connected you directly to God himself. Therefore, the potential for community exists with our brothers and sisters in Christ.

How we thrive best in life is where we have a sense of belonging and a sense of community. If we can't have community with our family of origin, then we build an extended family of friends, peers, and other persons who share our spiritual beliefs. Such a community has a purpose, and that purpose is to impact the societies and communities in which we live. Thus our sense of community spreads out from us and does not stop with us. It keeps us going. We have a sense of belonging that keeps us strong, supportive, and accountable so that we are the very best that we can be.

DL: What appears to me is that we build a community with people of like purposes and visions. For example, you can't build a community with someone who does not want to participate with you. Furthermore, when we build community with others, we draw out the best from our group members rather than competing with them.

EA: Here is an example, Dan. As your friend and encourager, I am trying to help you be the best seventh- and eighth-grade teacher you can be. I am encouraging you to be the best husband you can be, to be the best dad that you can be, to be the best person you can be. When we encourage each other in this manner, look at the world that we build.

DL: We build a world of hope.

EA: We not only build a world of hope, we build a world of accomplishment in which no one in the community we create will be hungry or experience major needs. All the major needs will be met in such a community. Love will be shared throughout that community. If we build communities on a small scale and these communities become more and more common, eventually we change the world.

Selfish Wealth: "Me, Myself, and I" at the Expense of Others and Community

EA: The purpose for our existence is not for ourselves. Our purpose is what we do in relationship to others. Unfortunately, we live in a culture that espouses a "me, myself, and I" philosophy. "It is what I do to get ahead." Such values propel a person to get his or her chunk of the American dream at the expense of others.

DL: There are plenty of people who chase down the American dream in the manner you have just described.

EA: Sure.

DL: All you have to do is look in the rich neighborhoods of our cities, see the size of the houses, and observe the preoccupation with wealth and status.

EA: It is the same here in Sun City West, Arizona. Your standing in the community is determined by the size of your home, the kind of car you drive, the clothes you wear, and the diamonds that you sport.

You have people who are the financial "cream of the crop" from other states who settle in places like Sun City West, Arizona. The values are transferred. You must have the big, powerful car. You must have more gold trim on your Cadillac than the other guy has. You must have the convertible or the Lincoln Continental with all the extras. You see gold-tinted wheel covers in the Safeway supermarket parking lot.

DL: I thought big cars were out, but apparently that is not the case in Sun City West.

EA: Big cars are in, and they are often driven by people who want to impress others.

DL: Is this everyone?

EA: No. There are some rich people who don't care and prefer to go shopping in their golf cart. The only difference might be if you have a pennant on your cart or a state flag that distinguishes your cart from the others.

DL: Moving on, I would like to explore now the approaches Powell advocates for achieving the goal of becoming a fully human, fully alive person. I don't want to explore all of these approaches. I prefer to discuss only those most significant to the theme of this book.

STRATEGIES FOR BECOMING FULLY HUMAN, FULLY ALIVE

A Confidant and Friend

DL: One of the most important things I see for achieving fullness and wholeness as a human being is having a confidant and friend. Powell [1976] states, "A person with whom we can be totally open is for many reasons an absolute requirement for growth into the fullness of life" [p. 115].

EA: If we dig into our background and our training and consider the ideals of our American heritage, which promote self-reliance and individualism, we are programmed to face life alone.

Now, self-reliance in and of itself is not a negative concept. We have to be independent in many ways. We have to take care of ourselves. We bear the responsibility of developing our gifts ourselves. Nevertheless, if I get to the point that I don't need others close to me to provide support, encouragement, and intimacy—if I get to the point that I believe that I am the captain of my own ship and others don't matter, then I am sailing on the *Titanic*, and I will hit an iceberg and sink.

I need you. I need others. We are connected to one another. We are brothers and sisters in the human experience whether we want to acknowledge that or not. I need people in my life.

I remember years ago that Donna and I were coming from some place in Northern California on our way back to Santa Cruz, California. As we approached San Francisco, we heard a disc jockey on our car radio announce the first release of Barbra Streisand's song, "People." You are familiar with the lyrics: "People who need people are the luckiest people in the world." In any case, the disc jockey played the record, and he said this at the conclusion: "That's a good song, if you need people." His implication was simple: "I don't need people. People are a hassle. I don't need them. I am a loner."

The loner is lonely because he needs people. Nevertheless, such a loner may be fearful that if he reaches out to others they will not meet his needs. Consequently, the loner doesn't try. He just gives up.

We need people. If you are to have an outward orientation, if you are to become a loving human being, there must be an object for that love. This object of love is whoever we encounter, be it a stranger, a person in need, or a neighbor. I cannot be a whole person without an object to love.

God and an Object of Love

EA: I think that is one reason why God is a Triune God. The Father must have an object. The Son must have an object. The Spirit must have an object. God loves the world; God loves the Son; it's that outward thing. The whole person is one who discovers what I just described and loves to love—just for the sake of loving and what that does for the other person. Love gets done.

Let Life Question You: A Second Look

DL: Let's move on to another step for achieving wholeness. I think this is one of the most important elements in Powell's proposals for a new life and a new vision based on the experiences I went through. Powell [1976] says we must be open and flexible and allow life to question us:

> You must believe with all your heart that you do not possess all truth in proper perspective. You must be ready to be questioned by life. Of course, every day, every event, and every person that touches your consciousness is questioning you. Do you love yourself? Can you enjoy yourself? What do you think of failure? Have you really recognized humanity and individuality in other people? Have you made the discovery of otherness? Do you like most people, or are they a bother? The first requirement to achieve a new life through a new vision is a readiness to hear and attempt to answer the questions that life will ask you. [p. 113]

So, Emil, even though we touched on this earlier in our discussion, what other thoughts do you have about this approach to fullness?

EA: Learning goes on for a lifetime. A person is always in the process of arriving at the goal of fullness and maturity. The process of learning in this life stops only when the Lord calls us home. It is then that the final changes will be made. We are growing, and we will be constantly growing.

There is no area in my life where I can say, "Okay, that is it; I have grown as far as I can." This is not true. I need always to be open to change and grow. My relationship with my wife, Donna, is in a growth mode. My relationship with you needs to be in a growth mode. I will *never* get to the point where I can say that I have grown enough. The day I do that is the day that I start dying. When my mind is fixed, and I don't have to change anymore, then I am in trouble.

Growth also comes in my reunderstanding of concepts. For example, there is the biblical truth that "God is love" [1 John 4:8, NIV]. I will never change this concept. Nevertheless, as I grow, I will change in my understanding of what this concept means.

DL: Your observation supports Powell's contention that we must be willing to be questioned by life and that we must be flexible enough to reframe our understanding of concepts and experiences. This is the ability to change. This ability to change and to be questioned by life includes the following principles, upon which we have already touched:

1. Every day, every event, and every person that touches your consciousness is questioning you.
2. We can learn to love and enjoy who we are.
3. Failure can be understood in new ways when we separate such a negative event from our personhood.
4. Humanity and individuality is to be celebrated in the lives of other people.

EA: I combine all of this into three goals: self-awareness, spontaneity, and intimacy.

For example, if I really know who I am, then I can be spontaneous with you. I don't have to stop, think, and say to myself, "Now, let's see. What should I say? How should I say this?" I can just be me and say what I want to say.

If I am guarded with people, I will be unauthentic. I will ask myself, "What do they want to hear from me so that they will like me?" This type of questioning illustrates that I don't know who I am. Awareness leads to spontaneity, and spontaneity opens the door to intimacy.

Sensory and Emotional Awareness

DL: What you have just described is partially illustrated in another approach Powell suggests to attaining fullness and wholeness in our human experience. Powell [1976] calls this "sensory and emotional awareness":

> It is necessary that you learn how to listen to your senses, and to register consciously the sights, sounds, smells, tastes, and touches of daily life. You will have to hear what your body is saying: when it is tired and when it is tense. This physical awareness is a prerequisite for emotional awareness because every emotion is a perceptual-physiological reality. In other words, an emotion exists partly in the mind and partly in the body. [p. 113]

One of the things I appreciated in the support you provided for me when I was going through the panic attacks was the affirmation that it was okay to *feel* what I was feeling in my moment of distress. In fact, instead of judging my feelings you have reaffirmed in our friendship that being in touch with my emotions is not only important but crucial to personal growth and intimacy. It is okay to respond to life. Our emotions are not wrong.

Another key in our dialogue has been understanding the difference between my adult self (big Dan) and the child self within (little Dan). I have the power to allow the adult Dan to respond to emotions and then make the appropriate choices. The little Dan does not have to be in control.

EA: One of the five freedoms of childhood is learning that our own feelings are okay. You and I grew up in homes where it wasn't okay for a child to have or own his or her feelings. For example, "Boys don't cry. You are supposed to be a big boy." Children are frequently discouraged from showing emotions with such reprimands as, "You shouldn't feel that way!"

Nevertheless, we do have feelings about things whether we are children or adults, and part of the fully human, fully alive experience is being able to own your feelings and understand them. Feelings are not right or wrong. When I experience a feeling, I can trace it back to a thought and address the origin of the thought. For example, I meet a person at church, and I am starting to feel uneasy. Why am I feeling uneasy? I start running back through my thoughts and discover that this person reminds me of someone who hurt me very deeply. My thoughts are, "Maybe I am going to get hurt again."

The Power of Thought Over the Fickleness of Feelings

This brings us to the next part of growth, which is the realization that I cannot live my life based on my feelings. The whole idea in transactional analysis with the development of the inner Adult, which begins at about ten months or so, is that a human begins to experience the ability to think. This thinking includes the ability to reason and to test reality. I can't live my life on the basis of my feelings. Feelings are fickle. Feelings can be influenced by what I ate, whether I am sick, whether I am tired, whether I am experiencing a chemical imbalance—whatever may be going on in my physical body. I have a mind; God gave me a mind. I need to learn how to use it. Consequently, any time I start to feel negatively about myself, I realize that the little child within me has been hooked. I need to be careful of this and not allow those feelings to control me.

The difficulty for most people is that feelings can be felt but thoughts are just thoughts. The question becomes, "How do I validate a thought?" Feelings are easy to validate because we experience their emotional impact. Children understand only what they can feel. The problem is that if such feelings are carried over into adulthood, the assumption is, "Anything I feel must be true." For example, if we feel something positive when we meet a potential life partner, we assume this has to be the person of our dreams because of our feelings. But where are the thoughts in all of this?

The apostle Paul says in Romans 12:2, "be transformed by the renewing of your mind" [NIV]. It is how we think that causes the way we live. Jesus said that it was out of the heart that the issues of life flow (Luke 6:45). The testing of reality with our thoughts frees us from inaccurate perceptions caused by our feelings.

THE RESTRUCTURING OF THOUGHT
AND VISION THERAPY

DL: Again, we are brought back again to Powell's restructuring of thought and his explanation of vision therapy [pp. 131-146].

EA: It is the whole rational approach. The Holy Spirit is the spirit of truth. The Holy Spirit does not come to the child of the parent; he comes to the adult. Christ appeals to the adult person. He doesn't deal with the feeling level or the prejudiced-talk level. He deals with reality. To say that the Holy Spirit is the spirit of truth is to say that the Holy Spirit is the spirit of reality. Christ comes as the *logos* (reason incarnate) and this is the essence of our thought process. The renewing of our thinking is where our wholeness lies.

The panic attack comes at the feeling level; it is not at the thinking level. The thinking is what allows the panic to come in and take over.

DL: We have been discussing the right to feel and the testing of reality with renewed thinking through the Adult self. How does this right to feel fit in with the rational process of a renewed vision and reframing of thoughts?

EA: The adult part of us can test reality and determine whether a feeling is valid. For example, consider the students you have worked with at the middle school. Some of those students respond to your teaching and you experience good feelings as a result. The adult in you says, "Dan, that is a legitimate feeling. Enjoy and celebrate the experience."

Nevertheless, you experience negative responses from other students, and your feelings tell you that you are a failure. In an appropriate response to these feelings, the adult self in you tests the reality and says, "Wait a minute. You are not a failure. Maybe what you are doing is failing, but *you* are not a failure. It is okay to feel bad about what is happening, but don't feel bad about being Dan Langford."

The testing of reality can legitimize your feelings about events that were not successful, and you have the right and the reason to feel disheartened because things did not work out as they were planned. Nevertheless, my discouragement should not project to my personhood. Feelings from negative outcomes do not give me the right to feel down about being *me*. I am still okay.

DL: You are separating the person and his or her inherent value from the negative circumstances.

EA: This is a separation of reality from delusion. To feel bad when something goes wrong is reality. To feel bad about being *me* is feeding back into the delusion of the little child (that archaic delusion), which says, "I have always been a failure. I will always be a failure."

When we separate who we are from what is happening to us is when no panic attack occurs. We may experience anxiety over what is happening to us in a particular situation, but no anxiety exists about who I am. This is the difference.

DL: I still cannot stand being closed in by a window seat on an airplane.

EA: That is a different thing.

DL: Yes, it is. According to Doctor Betat, who provided the medical help through my crisis, panic can be the result of a biochemical response [see Chapter 3]. He told the story of a patient of his who had no problem exploring caves when he was a teenager. However, when this person became older he developed an intolerance to wriggling through tight, closed-in spaces. When asked why the changes were happening, Doctor Betat suggested that chemical changes in this patient's brain may have caused him to become more claustrophobic as he got older. Doctor Betat further proposed that some fears we experience may be hereditary.

EA: The testing of reality with our thoughts could point to biochemical phenomena that may contribute to a panic response in certain situations. The key is to test reality and then allow the Holy Spirit to provide us with an honest assessment of what is happening to us.

Furthermore, supportive friends or groups can help us test reality. When we share our concerns with others and get input from others who are apart from the situation, such persons can give fresh perspectives and help the adult in us see things as they really are more clearly.

It Is Not a Pollyanna World

DL: In light of all we have discussed, Powell does not propose that we live in a Pollyanna world. Powell makes it clear that things happen to us which are not good. There are things in life which are very painful and, Powell [1976] puts it, "getting drunk on the raw liquor of Pollyannish hopes . . . is obvious and dangerous nonsense" [p. 43]. Hence, Powell [1976] argues:

It is obvious nonsense because changing one's thoughts about reality can change one's attitudes toward the facts but not the facts themselves. There is still grief over the death of a dear one. Failure still stings, and being overlooked still saddens. Of course, fully alive people will feel the "slings and arrows of outrageous fortune." They will grow into deeper, more sensitive, and more compassionate individuals precisely because they have suffered; but they will suffer. [pp. 43-44]

Suffering Has a Valuable Place in Life

EA: There is another aspect of this when we look into the writing of Thomas Merton and others. Suffering has a very valuable place in our lives. We don't go out and invite it into our experiences. We usually don't create it. It is a normal part of living as a human being. Consequently, some of the deepest and greatest lessons we learn are the ones that come through the times of testing. James 1:2 says this: "Consider it pure joy, my brothers, whenever you face trials of many kinds" [NIV].

I had a friend, younger than both of us, who just lost his wife. My friend is having a very difficult time going through the process of losing his wife. Even though this individual (a long-time Christian friend) is a psychotherapist, he is absolutely devastated.

I shared an e-mail with him the other day, and I wrote, "You need to know that as you walk through this valley, the Lord is going to give back to you a person you never were before this happened. You will become a person you could never have been apart from this experience."

So, when we look at tragedy, trouble, and suffering, as I said earlier, the question is not "Why me?" but "What am I going to learn? What am I going to discover?" The suffering will either make you or break you. You will either end up as a bitter human being, angry at God and at life, or you will be a therapist (healer) who has become more sensitive than he or she has ever been in life.

My friend is three months into the process, and he is beginning to see changes in his life that I have just described.

Chapter 11

Finale: Relational Theology and the Circle of Life

Emil Authelet

INTRODUCTION

The Primal Boundaries of the World Are Natural

When humankind began walking in space, it became obvious from that perspective that no boundaries mark the borders of countries except for bodies of water and geographical landmarks. The only human-made boundary visible to the naked eye from space is the Great Wall of China. Consequently, most human-made boundaries are invisible, yet those are the boundaries that separate territories and nations. Likewise, we construct other boundaries to separate ourselves from others—these too are human-made and maintained. As with psychological games, the purpose of such walls—such boundaries— is to avoid closeness, involvement, and intimacy.

Doing Away with Boundaries That Separate: Biblical Illustrations

In contrast, the New Testament speaks of doing away with the old, human-made boundaries. The apostle Paul wrote of the removal of these borders in his letter to the Galatians. Gone were the divisions between male or female, slave or free, those in and those out, or any other distinction created for the purpose of closing out, keeping out, or rubbing out others. Paul declared that we, as believers in Christ, are all one—members one of another—not simply because we are all part of a single race—the human race—but because we are all created in a single image (see Galatians 3:26-28, NIV).

Extending Paul's idea of the oneness of Christian believers, a parallel application can be made to all of us who are a part of the human family. You are part of me; I am part of you. We are part with those who were, are today, and will yet be—for time is another artificial barrier we construct. Similarly, what happens to me also happens to you; what happens to you happens to me. There is but one source of life, and we all partake of that source.

The Hazard of Rugged Individualism

Nevertheless, because of our fear, insecurity, and anxiety, many of us have turned away from the principles of oneness and community. Instead, we have bought into a theory of "rugged individualism." "Rugged individualism" fits with the unhealthy self-perceptions of the Inner Child who maintains that winning is everything. You know how those sayings go: The one with the most toys wins. Get before you are gotten. The emphasis is on achievement, accumulating, and attaining the enviable status of being number one. So, we love things, use people, seek to get ahead regardless of the cost, develop disposable relationships, and trust no one.

All of this feeds into our fears; it also *feeds* our fears. When have we ever won enough, accumulated enough, achieved enough, and at the same time found some sense of meaning in it all?

Believing in "rugged individualism" means everyone else is our competitor, for only so much exists to go around, and not everyone can be number one in everything. Furthermore, when our abilities are limited, as everyone's are, how do we compensate in such a competitive world?

Everyone wants a piece of the "Great American Dream" (to achieve, accumulate, and be number one), which every free Adult knows is a delusion. Nevertheless, this is not understood by the Inner Child, who still believes in fairy tales. Not everyone can be billionaire or possess a billion of anything—except maybe bills. Yet the belief persists that anyone can be a top dog: "If he did it, so can I!"

Nevertheless, let's suppose we do become top dogs. So what? What do you really have? These dreams further isolate us from others because they stand in the way of our real dream, which is to be loved.

Boundaries of Fear and Anxiety Separate Us from One Another

Boundaries we construct out of fear and anxiety separate us from one another, when in reality what we really want most is to be loved. In absence of love, we seek to replace it with achievements, accumulation, and activities. We are human beings, not human doings; doing can never substitute for being. Nonetheless, human doing drives the Inner Child, who is so afraid that he or she is incapable of being loved that the Inner Child isolates himself or herself through doing and expecting others to do for her or him. The Inner Child says, "You make me happy." "You do for me what I cannot do for myself." "Love me!" "Make me feel I'm worth loving."

The Will to Relate

Freud saw the basic need of life as "the will to pleasure." Adler saw it as "the will to power." Jung saw it more as "the will to 'authentic being'." Viktor Frankl, after his experience in a Nazi concentration camp, saw it as "the will to meaning." Robert Schuller (1982), in his book, *Self-Esteem: The Second Reformation,* saw it as "the will to self-esteem." Much of pop psychology agrees with Schuller. Like various facets of a diamond, each of these interpreters has an insight that is part of a whole, yet the whole is more than the sum of its parts.

In the Hebrew Bible and also in the Christian New Testament, God sums up the basic human need in life as, "the will to relate." To rephrase the concept, the outworking of this "will to relate" means that a person is in harmony with God, others, self, life, and the created order. It is "the will to love and be loved." Within this is pleasure, true power, authentic being, meaning, self-esteem, and so much more based on harmony with God, others, self, and life. This is what it means to be fully human, fully alive!

Our Physical and Spiritual Dualism

We are not just flesh and blood in our makeup as human beings. We are more than our physical origin of conception and the life that has evolved from that accidental beginning. We are spiritual beings, created in the image of a Triune God, who is love. We are spiritual beings made for love and capable of loving. We are spiritual beings, created within a spiritual image, for a spiritual purpose, on a spiritual mission, with a spiritual power, to achieve a spiritual end, in a spiritual way, to glorify God. We come from God; we move, live, and have our being in God; we will return to God when this physical pilgrimage ends to live with our Creator-Friend forever. Consequently, we have one Lord, one essence, one life, one destiny, and must live as one with Him and with each other.

How each of us lives out this journey as a physical being with a spiritual dimension affects all others around us as they impact us. This is why Jesus' prayer for us is that we may be one, as He and the Father are one (John 17:20-21). Therefore, our caregiving and, more specifically, Christian caregiving, must fit within this divine model. This is the model Jesus lived for us. He is our example as well as our enablement. We are to pattern our approach after the Jesus model.

Made for Loving and the Problem of Alienation

We as human beings also share a single purpose. We are made for love and loving. That is why we cannot stand alienation. It is contrary to our nature. Alienation affects us mentally, socially, emotionally, sexually, psychologically, spiritually, relationally, and physically. It is the most destructive force in our inner lives as well as within our bodies. Not only are we affected by it, but we also affect others when we are out of harmony with them. When seen on a world scale, what we have is a world gradually self-destructing because of alienation— separated from those we have offended, those who have offended us, and those we have not even come to know but have chosen to neglect, for whatever reason. We are against the world; the world is against itself. To be against another is to be against the self. The only way healing can be present is when we choose to love all others.

Most of the ills in this world are traceable to alienation. The story of Adam and Eve in the third chapter of Genesis, is the archetype of this problem. Verse 23 describes what happened as a result of the disobedience that alienated Adam and Eve from God:

> So the Lord banished him from the Garden of Eden to work the ground from which he had been taken. After he drove the man out, he placed on the east side of the Garden of Eden cherubim

and a flaming sword flashing back and forth to guard the way to the tree of life. (Genesis 3:23-24, NIV)

We are what we are, depending on who has loved us and who has not. Since we did not choose our parents, many of us grew up with some heavy loads to bear. Others of us had a wonderful beginning because we were made to feel loved, affirmed, and special. A few of us were so wounded by an absence of love that we didn't even recognize the problem until later on when love became evident in our lives.

We are made for love, but somehow, for some of us, those upon whom we depended for love didn't get the message, probably because others before them never got that message either. Maybe now we can begin to understand why God made loving Him, others, and self a command!

THINKING AND RELATING HOLISTICALLY

Community and Identity in Primitive Society

Many primitive societies on earth retain individual identity within a model of community. In these primitive societies, a person's identity is meaningless apart from the nuclear family, extended family, and community. However, within industrialized nations, the pressures of production and profit coupled with urbanization have resulted in the ideals of community being replaced with the ideals of individuality and the attendant pathologies. To make a transition from a paradigm of individuality to a paradigm of community is very difficult in our modern society. Nevertheless, it is within the paradigm of community that the salvation of humanity is found.

Tensions Between Concepts of Community and Individuality

Despite the good in a community paradigm, if such a model is perceived by the rest of the world as hostile and competitive with the status quo of individuality, any effort to bring about community is limited and bound to the "birds of a feather" who share the vision.

When the predominant model of a society is individuality, this individuality comes with presuppositions and assumptions that minimize the need for community. Worst of all, individuality creates a sense of pride and smugness that deepens the alienation. This is often why individuality lacks meaning in the deepest sense. No ultimate meaning exists in personal and material gain that isolates a person from others. The paradigm of individuality does not work for spiritual beings possessed of a will to relate. The will to relate is our basic essence. To deny that is to self-destruct.

From smaller communities—the nuclear family, the extended family, and culture—emerges the recognition of the larger context, nations, and the world. The world community is our family. However, to own this as reality means to radically rethink our individualism and all the evils it represents. Many know the seriousness of these problems intellectually but do not know how to resolve the dilemmas practically. Nevertheless, until a practical resolution occurs to problems inherent in the paradigm of individualism, nothing will really change.

Change Is Needed: Think in Terms of Community Instead of Individuality

We have known theologically for centuries that change needs to happen. But recognizing the need for change has failed to affect the way we live. Sunday morning at 11:00 is still the most segregated hour in American life. In another context, less than 20 percent of the population of the world consumes more than half of the world's goods. How can one nation have such a high standard of living while much of the rest of the world struggles to subsist? What theology can account for this?

Theology and the Philosophical Framework

Centuries ago, when theology was draped on a philosophical framework, it was not person centered. Desperately needed was a psychological framework, but that was not to come until the twentieth century. Even today, theology on a psychological framework still struggles for acceptance. We are relational beings, desperately in need of a relational theology that encompasses the entire human race as well as God and self.

Theology Draped Over a Psychological/Relational Framework

Our worldview, in order to fit reality, must see race as a whole, responsibility as universal, and the potential for love and being loved as realizable. Only this larger context fits reality. Only this larger context fits our true need. Philosophical and scientific paradigm shifts seem to precede theological shifts because it is so hard for theological paradigms to change—even though the biblical witness is clearly present. The tail wags the dog. Theology should have set the pace and determined the way. This cannot happen when theology is divorced from life, much less from the Word of God. The history of Israel and Christianity fell pray to the same delusion: "God sees us as special and the rest are just the rest." Attitudes within religious institutions have been like those of kids who just completed building their tree house. The first thing those kids want to do is pull up the rope so that no one else can get in.

Humankind Is a Totality

Humankind is one, a totality, whether we want to recognize it or not. This totality of humankind is as clear as John 3:16 and God's love for the world. God loves the whole wide world. This is the world for which Christ died and for which God offers His grace and love. This is the world He commands us to love. This is the world we are to evangelize with His love, forgiveness, and reconciliation.

This is the world we are a part of, no matter what artificial barriers we may seek to construct. This is also the world for which we are held responsible by Him in the judgment to come. To have any other worldview is to be antichrist, to be un-Christian. It is the only world Jesus Christ knows, and to partake of him is to partake of his mission for that world.

Matthew 25:31-40 presents this reality to us:

> When the Son of Man comes in his glory, and all the angels with him, he will sit on his throne in heavenly glory. All the nations will be gathered before him, and he will separate the people one from another as a shepherd separates the sheep from the goats. He will put the sheep on his right and the goats on his left.

Then the King will say to those on his right, "Come, you who are blessed by my Father; take your inheritance, the kingdom prepared for you since the creation of the world. For I was hungry and you gave me something to eat, I was thirsty and you gave me something to drink, I was a stranger and you invited me in, I needed clothes and you clothed me, I was sick and you looked after me, I was in prison and you came to visit me."

Then the righteous will answer him, "Lord, when did we see you hungry and feed you, or thirsty and give you something to drink? When did we see you a stranger and invite you in, or needing clothes and clothe you? When did we see you sick or in prison and go to visit you?"

The King will reply, "I tell you the truth, whatever you did for one of the least of these brothers of mine, you did for me." (NIV)

CHRISTOLOGY

My Commitment to the Christian Faith Has Created My Worldview

As a person who believes in the redemptive power of Christ, I contend because of my faith that the redemptive power of Christ as understood in the New Testament is the only hope for humankind (see John 14:6). If we are unable to accept and celebrate this truth, it is because we do not really understand the New Testament writings, nor do we understand what it means to be spiritually and experientially connected to the personhood and love of Christ.

Writings found especially in the Gospel of John and Paul's letter to the Romans declare not only that Christ is God in the flesh, but also that Christ, as God in the flesh, died for all humankind (see John 1 and Romans 5).

To embrace this faith I have just described, the faithful are challenged to embrace the same concern and love for others that is exhibited in the life and teachings of Christ. 2 Peter 3:9b states, "He [the Lord] is patient with you, not wanting anyone to perish, but everyone to come to repentance" (NIV). Wouldn't it be nice if we were also that willing? Thus, the wellness and wholeness of the entire world is to be our concern. Whatever is in the heart of Christ needs to be in our hearts as well.

Superficial Faith

Many of us as professing Christians have allowed ourselves to gravitate into a familiarity with the superficialities of our faith which have bred contempt. We actually think we can be Christian without living as a Christian! We believe we can live in the world God created as his own and not be mutually responsible to assist in changing what God sent his Son to change. Redemption happens privately, but redemption is no private matter. Contrary to what happened on the *Titanic*, we can't lock the third-class passengers below decks and save the glory-bound lifeboats for ourselves. The arrogance of this is against everything that God is about.

Self-Serving Attitudes

The self-serving attitudes of society and politics of the United States typify this arrogance. The following are examples of these attitudes:

- Save Kuwait because we need the oil and its profits.
- Ignore Angola because it has no strategic value within our economy.

Is one human being of more value than another? Certainly not to God.

GOD'S ORIGINAL INTENTION
AND OUR DEEPEST NEED

To understand God's original intention as well as our deepest need, we must define again who we are, why we are here, and what this journey is all about:

We are spiritual beings,
Fashioned in the image of a Spiritual Being—
The Triune God
Sent to live a spiritual life
In a spiritual way
Within a spiritual realm
For a spiritual purpose

To a spiritual end
By a spiritual means

To the glory of God
And to our own personal joy.

Spiritual Unity Was Marred by Rebellion

God's original intention for humankind was marred by the entrance of rebellion against God (Genesis 3) but fully restored by the redemptive work of Jesus Christ (Romans 5:15-20). Hence, God's plan for humankind is that we are to live in harmony with the Triune God, with all others, ourselves, and life within His specially created order.

Humans Are Relational Beings

Since we have been fashioned in the image of God (Genesis 1:26-27), God fashioned us as relational beings, created to enjoy Him and His world fully, and to enjoy living in harmony with self and all others. Every major concept in the Hebrew Bible and Christian New Testament is relational. Love is relational, as is justice, mercy, peace, atonement, and other Hebrew concepts. Concurrently, New Testament terms such as grace, forgiveness, reconciliation, redemption, peace, love, and mercy are relational terms. The relationships are between us and God, others, our true selves, and life itself. The Christian life is to be lived in these harmonious relationships—to fail to do so is to fail to be Christian. All that God has done for us in Christ is relational. The purpose has been to bring us back into harmony with God, others, self, and life. We are to love God with all our being and to love others as we love ourselves. This is the life Christ came to establish in reconciling us to Himself. This is the life He instills within each believer re-creating us as His friends and then lovers of all humankind. God knows that our deepest need is give love rather than just be loved. However, we can never learn this until we become immersed within His unconditional love for us. Once we are in harmony with God, and our eyes are opened to His vision, we begin to discover our deepest need is not to be loved; it is to be loving.

Love Is Outward

Again, as documented in John 3:16, the orientation of love is outward. "God so loved that He gave . . ." To be loved is wonderful—beyond measure. Nevertheless, to be loving is the *great joy* of life in Christ. It is Christ's love flowing out through us to others in their real needs that fulfills the deepest need in us, which is loving others. It is God revealing Himself in and through us, to others.

1 John 4:7 declares the source of love: "Dear friends, let us love one another, for love comes from God. Everyone who loves has been born of God and knows God" (NIV). The same chapter also reveals to us God's basic essence—He is love. God only loves. This is who He is.

Anyone re-created in the image of Christ because of a choice to connect with Christ is also made for love. We know we are His—we are of Him—because of loving others. The Fruit of the Spirit (Galatians 5:22,23) as well as the essence of 1 Corinthians 13 is this love for others. We are God lovers and we are lovers of others in His Name. This is our deepest need. Here is where we find purpose, meaning, fulfillment, and a lasting sense of joy.

If we are stuck within our need to be loved instead of loving, such a condition is evidence of our need for healing and wholeness. As we heal, the orientation shifts from self to others. The flow becomes outward. We see this in the writings of Jeremiah, Ezekiel, and Isaiah as well as within the New Testament and especially with Jesus in the Gospels. Out of us as healers and lovers come rivers of living water.

This is also the New Testament picture of the disciple or follower of Christ. Like Abraham of old, we are to be a blessing to all other nations—all other people. God's redemption is universal; it is offered to all. We as lovers and healers are given a similar challenge: Love always demands an object. Our object of love is God's entire world.

Caregiving: A Way of Life for Believers

Caregiving is a way of life for the believer. Caregiving is how one participates in the Kingdom of God. God's kingdom is a kingdom of love. It is also a kingdom of lovers, sharing His love and good news with all humankind. The kin of the kingdom are those called to share God's love with his entire world. Remember the lyrics to the old Sunday school song, "red and yellow, black and white, all are precious in His sight." All of humankind is included. Further, our priorities in reaching out to those around us should be the same triage exhibited by Christ: serve the most needy first.

Caregiving for God's world takes on many forms, but it is the primary calling of the "called-out ones" or the church universal. To truly participate with God is to participate in His mission. This makes us God's caregivers, accountable to Him and to His world. We could have no greater or more rewarding task.

THE MUTUAL INTERCONNECTEDNESS BETWEEN THERAPIST AND CLIENT

The Therapist and Client Are One

In the therapeutic relationship, the therapist and client are one. This is the reality of the relationship, whether or not the therapist and client have this understanding.

Failure to understand the oneness between the therapist and client blocks real healing and lets us know that hidden agendas need to be dealt with for the relationship to be what it needs to be. True healing requires a full recognition of this reality. It works in both directions.

The Relationship of Therapist to Client

How the client is perceived by the therapist is foundational to the healing process. As stated earlier, it is to be like Buber's "I-Thou." I'm not here to fix you, as if I am some psychological mechanic, but I can enter your pain with you and help you explore ways out. We are in this together. You have trusted me with your pain and I am trusting you to do your work to move through it into full healing.

The Relationship of Client to Therapist

How the therapist is perceived by the client may be faulty unless the therapist provides input. The therapist will challenge the perceptions of the client until reality becomes accepted. Most clients have been preconditioned toward a "fix me" attitude of expectations, such as within the medical profession; however, true healing requires clients to learn how to take charge of their own healing. The clients are there to work on their pain, to find realistic and meaningful options for dealing with it, and to learn how to work through it as needed, while moving away from earlier forms of dealing with it. The therapist is there for the client; the client is there for his or her own sake and well-being. They are working through the pain because that is the right thing to do.

Person to Person

When both the therapist and client are able to meet as equals, then the healing process has truly begun. The ability to meet as equals cements the foundation for the therapeutic relationship. Many therapists are unable to achieve this because of their own unmet needs. Clients may be unable to achieve this because of preconceived notions regarding the therapist and therapy, as well as because of the insecurities of the therapist.

The brokenness of the client is based in past alienations and inadequate forms of relating. The client has developed certain ways of relating to deal with the inner pathology, which only perpetuate the inner pain. The interconnectedness between therapist and client must now speak to this faulty way of relating and challenge it with reality and healing. The healing takes place within this relationship. Perhaps for the first time the client experiences what it is like to be in a loving, caring, redemptive relationship. This growth and healing comes for the client when the client is able to connect to the health, wholeness, and unconditional love within the therapist. As a result, the client can be free to work on his or her healing. The foundation has been set. The building of a new life can now take place.

A Triune Relationship

God is the Healer, the therapist is His agent/caregiver, and the client appropriates the healing offered by the Healer. The caregiver is helping meet the real need of the client by allowing the client to encounter reality and to learn to reality-test one's thinking, feeling, and acting and, in this process, discover true life and living. Without this relating, the client would most likely be unable to experience a genuine, loving, and caring form of relating.

I remember working with Marilyn years ago. She was referred to me by her family physician. A few sessions after meaningful changes had occured for her, she felt she had gained enough new insights to go it on her own. Some weeks later when I saw her physician, he told me of her changes and her new outlook on life. When he asked her what I had done for her, she had reflected for a moment, and then answered accordingly:

> First, I felt totally accepted as I am. The other thing was, he listened. Just being listened to made me feel like a worthwhile person who had sense enough to know what she needed to do to get her life back on track.

Marilyn later became a caregiver within her church's caregiving program. What those with whom she worked appreciated most about her was her ability to listen. True listening takes place between equals. Since we are relational beings and our dysfunctioning results from poor or inadequate relationships, healing comes through adequate and meaningful ways of relating. To state it again for emphasis, healing is within the relationship. The caregiver, as the "wounded healer," enters the relationship to be a healing agent, allowing God to bring healing to the one in need. God is committed to the process for the ongoing healing and maturing of therapist and client. This takes place within the triangle of Healer, therapist, and client—the true healing relationship.

AUTHENTIC CAREGIVING

The Extension of Self for the Well-Being of the Other

Authentic caregiving takes place within the extension of the self for the well-being of the other. M. Scott Peck (1978) sees this as a definition of love (see also Peck, 1993). Howard Clinebell has a similar conclusion: it is a need-satisfying relationship in a dependable way.[1] In both, the caregiver extends herself or himself on behalf of another for that person's well-being and does it dependably, day after day, experience after experience. This is the way it is. An illustration of this perpetuity is found in Hebrews 13:8: "Jesus Christ is the same yesterday, today, and forever" (NIV). This perpetuity ideally becomes the model for the caring therapist. The therapist says, "I am here to be with you today in your need; I will be here as long as needed. I will not leave you unattended. I am here for you."

Life-Gifting to the Other

This way of relating and the quality of the relationship shared is a life-gifting of one to the other. It is a way of relating that the person receiving care may have never experienced before. It brings life to the recipient. It is a new birth. It is a giving of what may have been missing or was only present minimally during formative years, depriving the Inner Child of what she or he truly needed for a sense of self-worth and meaning. Now it is being shared in full measure and the inner Adult is able to respond to it in life-changing ways. This is what caregiving is all about.

My relationship with Dan has been a love-gift to him with the acceptance, approval, and affirmation he needed to firm up his psychological muscles so that he could cope with rejection, disappointment, and possible failure as they really are and not internalize them and put the blame and shame on himself, like little Dan wanted to do. It was to allow Dan to see himself through my eyes and not the eyes of little Dan, whose vision was badly distorted due to earlier life experiences. My offer of care was to hold up a new mirror to Dan, the Adult, a mirror of reality testing, that showed him what he really is: capable, caring, a wonderful spiritual being, the apple of God's eye. Seeing this truth—sensing this and in time learning to feel it—forced Dan to change his way of thinking about himself and about the events he has struggled with. He has learned that "Even if you fail, you are not a failure! You are worth loving."

BUILDING A WORLD OF CAREGIVERS

Am I My Brother's Keeper?

Cain raised the question that we must learn not only to answer but also learn how to fulfill in today's declining world: "Am I my brother's keeper?" (Genesis 4:9b). Yes, we are the other person's keeper, because we are brothers and sisters to all others. Every person is a spiritual being who is a part of the whole, and the whole is responsible for the part—every single, solitary part. Artificial boundaries are just that; they have no place within reality. To write off any part of the whole is to help destroy the whole.

Genocide in Africa, a nuclear disaster in the Ukraine contaminating lives, violence in Northern Ireland, domestic abuse in our neighborhoods—all are linked and intertwined. They all involve people whom God loves. We are to love them, too. How to love all of God's people may be another question that needs resolution. Facing responsibility for other human beings cannot be debated. We must care for the whole; to show that care, we must build a world of caregivers who genuinely care.

Love Cannot Tolerate a World of Opulence Alongside Dire Poverty

Love cannot tolerate a planet where one is stuffed and 100 others are starving. Love cannot tolerate life in which the "have-nots" far outnumber the "haves," and the "have-lots" are increasing daily at the expense of the "haves" and "have-nots." Love cannot tolerate an environment being pillaged for the benefit of the "have-lots" when they steal from the "have-nots" the very quality of the air they breathe.

God has not created a privileged class to indulge themselves; God gave wealth to the "haves" to enable them to care for the "have-nots" so that none would perish because of need. Our contempt for God is expressed when we refuse to give and show love to the world around us. We were created to be lovers and givers. To do less corporately is to seal the doom of the human species.

The Price of Being Selfish

When we are selfish, unloving, and ungiving, we pollute our own homes, destroy our own futures, and guarantee our children's children will inherit a world unfit for their real needs. We have the ability, now, to meet the world's true needs; it is the sharing first of our hearts and then of life's abundance.

WHAT IS HEALTH?

The Disease Model

Psychology is well acquainted with pathology, just as the field of medicine is. Nevertheless, defining wholeness and wellness is another matter altogether for these disciplines. Theology has its struggles here as well. Philosophy has done a better job, but still the field needs further defining. Powell (1976) describes what it is to be "fully human, fully alive," but what does it mean to be fully spiritual, fully mature, fully in harmony with God, others, self, and life? That must be our focus. That is the source of our true meaning and purpose. This is true emotional and spiritual health.

Relational Health

Relational health is the ability to establish and maintain healthy forms of relating with God, others, self, and life—to the glory of God. It is to live in harmony at all these levels. The antithesis is to perceive oneself to be in harmony with God while alienated from others. The antithesis of true harmony is to live a delusion of what health and wholeness really mean.

Furthermore, to live in isolation within a safe context, such as one's own little community or culture or world to the point of ignoring those outside the comfort zone, is also delusional. The context of health is all humankind, just as the God/Other/Self/Life Relationship includes all humankind.

Coming to wholeness, meaning, purpose, and mission are all parts of this holistic approach of thinking, relating, and living. Thus, health is more than the absence of sickness and alienation. One is never free of disease or unease. The truth is, disease is ubiquitous, and disease is held in check, physically, by a healthy immune system and emotionally by a vibrant philosophy of life that holds it together through thick and thin.

A Healthy Philosophy of Life

What is a healthy philosophy of life? Here are some of the characteristics:

1. It has within it all the basic qualities of maturity. Its focus is on being, not doing.
2. A good philosophy of life manifests good levels of self-esteem, self-worth, self-acceptance, and meaningful levels of self-giving.
3. For the Christian, a good philosophy of life is growing up into the full maturity Christ intended. It is a spiritual direction in which the person is actively and intentionally involved in a God-invited process of maturing up into Christ for others, to the glory of God. We are in it for Him and for others (Ephesians 4:11-16).

To become all God intended us to become in relationship to God/Others/Self/Creation is a lifelong process demanding everything of the pilgrim/seeker. Yet no true health exists apart from involvement in this process. This process is really what life is and how it is to be lived. This is the calling of the caregiver as well as of all humankind. This is what we all should be about. We are to bring the whole of humanity along this same journey. The issue is not whether we gain followers. The issue is that this is the calling chosen by God for caring and believing human beings.

THE RESPONSIBILITY OF THE THERAPIST

Healing Takes Place in Relationship

Healing takes place within the context of relationship. Therefore, what the therapist brings to the relationship is essential. For this reason, the therapist needs to be all she or he can be as a person as well as a skilled clinician. It means dealing with one's own issues so as to be the best partner one can be with the client and to be in tune to the client's real needs. Like in any meaningful relationship, such as parent to child, therapist to client, doctor to patient, person to person, each needs to be all they can be for the sake of the other. To assist a client to come to awareness, spontaneity, and intimacy, the therapist in partnership with client needs to facilitate the best from both of them in the process. Consequently, the greater burden for modeling what needs to be in place resides with the professional caregiver. Out of this style of relating, the client is encouraged to achieve his or her best as well.

The Therapist's Ongoing Journey to Wholeness

To be a facilitator of wholeness and relational health necessitates an ongoing journey in wholeness for the therapist. Such growth is a lifelong process. The emerging growth within the client provokes new growth within the therapist. As a result, the therapist shares out of that growth as an encouragement to the client's growth. The process is mutually need satisfying. This growth is also evidence that the relationship is working. God is at work here.

To model wholeness and relational health is no easy task, especially in times of one's own deep needs born of stress, crisis, and trauma. At those times, one is called upon to model how to handle stress, crisis, and trauma and, in time, to give evidence of how one can succeed. The process is never completed as long as life lasts. To be in process is our calling, and the assurance that the process continues is our major focus. Nonetheless, the results are in God's hands. Our being is still in the process of becoming. We are not yet all we shall be, but at the same time we are far more than we once were when the journey began. The free Adult within the therapist is entering into and assisting the hurt, pain, and loss of the client. No matter how long this process may take, the result is the freedom of the client to become what he or she is destined to become. Therapists love clients enough to meet and accept them where they are, but also not to leave them there and instead encourage maturity.

Advocating for the Wholeness and Relational Health of All Humankind

The other responsibility of the therapist is to advocate for wholeness and relational health for all humankind. This begins in one's present context. What are the causes of stress, crisis, and trauma in life? Why do so many persons grow up with dysfunctional problems? Why are there so many problems with crime and abuse and brokenness? Why is there so much sin?

Our task is threefold:

1. To understand the past and to help persons attain release from its tyranny

2. To broaden our understanding of health and its meaning in the present for the sake of all humankind
3. To heal the future through the providing of all that is necessary for discovering and experiencing full life in Christ at this moment in time

A Caregiving World

To do all of this we need a caregiving world with caregivers willing to spend and be spent for the glory of God. God loves caregivers. God also loves all those needing their care. Thus, His command is that we are to extend ourselves for the well-being of others.[2]

To do all of this we need a caregiving world with caregivers willing to spend and be spent for the glory of God. God loves caregivers. He is one Himself. God also loves all those needing care, that is why He has commissioned so many caregivers. Thus, His command is that we are to extend ourselves for the well-being of others.

Can you imagine a world in which the example of Jesus Christ is being lived out by all those who name His Name so that His world is receiving the love and caregiving it so deeply needs and deserves? A world in which real needs are felt and met. A world in which caregivers get care when needed. A world in which patients become whole and they in turn learn to care for others. A world in which people are both loved and loving.

Welcome to God's Kingdom of Love!

Notes

Chapter 4

1. The term relational theology refers to a theology constructed on a biblical psychology rather than a traditional approach to philosophy as seen in historic theological constructs.

2. The terms Inner Child, Parent, and Adult, found in transactional analysis, were first encountered by me in the writing of Dr. Hugh Missildine (1963) in his book *Your Inner Child of the Past.*

3. Shame is always a major component when the Inner Child is in control and is facing the fear of failure.

Chapter 7

1. I have encouraged my friend to journal his daily journey in completing his grief process and recovery, then to write about it for both clients and caregivers to read and experience. As a skilled caregiver and a highly esteemed colleague within the profession, his experience needs to be shared.

2. For information about an excellent lay-caregiving program, *The Stephen Ministries,* founded by Dr. Kenneth Haugk, contact: Stephen Ministries, 8016 Dale, St. Louis, MO 63117-1449. It should be in place in every local church.

Chapter 11

1. From class notes and discussion with Dr. Howard Clinebell, Professor of Pastoral Care and Counseling, Claremont School of Theology, Claremont, CA, 1964-1965.

2. Three major sources for further consideration: *Testaments of Love: A Study of Love in the Bible,* by Leon Morris (Eerdmans: Grand Rapids, 1981; especially Chapters 7 through 11, and the conclusion); *The Love Command in the New Testament,* by Victor Paul Furnish (Abingdon: Nashville, 1972; especially Chapters 1, 4, 5, and the conclusion); *On Love,* by Pierre Teilhard de Chardin (Collins: St. James Place, London, 1972).

Bibliography

Agras, W. S. (1985). *Panic: Facing fears, phobias, and anxiety.* New York: W. H. Freeman.

American Psychiatric Association (1994). *Diagnostic and statistical manual of mental disorders,* Fourth edition. Washington, DC.

American Psychological Association (2000). Answers to your questions about panic disorder. APA Public Communications [online]. Available online at: <http://www.apa.org/pubinfo/panic/.html>.

Arndt, W.F. and Gingrich, F.W. (1979). *A Greek-English lexicon of the New Testament and other early Christian literature.* Chicago: University of Chicago Press.

Barclay, W. (1975a). The letters of James and Peter. In W. Barclay (Ed.), *The daily study Bible series* (pp. 130-132). Philadelphia: Westminster.

Barclay, W. (1975b). The letters to the Corinthians. In W. Barclay (Ed.), *The daily study Bible series* (pp. 169-171). Philadelphia: Westminster.

Barlow, D.H. (1990). Long-term outcome for patients with panic disorder treated with cognitive-behavioral therapy. *Journal of Clinical Psychiatry,* 51(12, Suppl. A), 17-23.

Barlow, D.H. (1992). Cognitive-behavioral approaches to panic disorder and social phobia. *Bulletin of the Menninger Clinic* [online], Spring 92 Suppl. 56(2). Available online at: <http://ehostvgw2.epnet.com/delivery.asp?d...der&startHitNum =1&rlStartHit=1&delType=FT>.

Barlow, D.H. and Bufka, L.F. (1999). Anxiety. In *Microsoft Encarta Encyclopedia 99* (pp. 1-7). [CD-ROM]. (1993-1998). Microsoft Corporation.

Berne, E. (1964). *The psychology of human relationships.* New York: Grove Press.

Berne, E. (1977). *Intuition and ego states: The origins of transactional analysis.* San Francisco: T.A. Press.

Bradshaw, J. (1988). *Healing the shame that binds you.* Deerfield Beach, FL: Health Communications.

Bradshaw, J. (1992). *Homecoming: Reclaiming and championing your inner child.* New York: Bantam, Doubleday, Dell Publishers.

Brown, A. and Lempa, M. (2000). Update on potential causes and new treatments for anxiety disorders. *NARSAD Research.* Available online at: <http://www. mhsource.com/narsad/anxiety.html>.

Cadieux, R.J. (1996). Azapirones: An alternative to benzodiazepines for anxiety. *American Family Physician* [online], 53(7). Available online at: <http://web7. infotrac.galegroup.com/itw/in . . . _0_A18364663&dyn=7!ar_fmt?sw_aep= uphoenix>.

Chambers, O. (1936/1955). *So send I you.* Grand Rapids, MI: Discovery House Publishers.

Collins, G. R. (1981). *Psychology and theology.* Nashville: Abingdon.

Crabb, L. (1997). *Connecting: Healing for ourselves and our relationships: A radical new vision.* Nashville: Word.

Craske, M.G., Brown, T.A., and Barlow, D.H. (1991). Behavioral treatment of panic disorder: A two year follow-up. *Behavioral Therapy, 22,* 289-304.

Crowe, R.R. (1990). Molecular genetics and panic disorder: New approaches to an old problem. In J.C. Ballenger (Ed.), *Neurobiology of panic disorder, Volume 8: Frontiers of clinical neuroscience* (pp. 59-70). New York: Wiley-liss.

Cully, I.V. (1984). *Education for spiritual growth.* San Francisco: Harper and Row.

David, H. (1970). *What the world needs now, and other love lyrics.* New York: Trident Press.

Erikson, E. (1982). *The life cycle completed.* New York: Norton.

Faravelli, C. (1985). Life events preceding the onset of panic disorder. *Journal of Affective Disorders, 1,* 103-105.

Farmer, S. (1990). *Adult children of abusive parents: A healing program for those who have been physically, sexually, or emotionally abused.* New York: Ballantine.

Forward, S. and B. Craig (1988). *Betrayal of innocence: Incest and its devastation.* New York: Penguin.

Fossum, M. and Mason, M. (1986). *Facing shame.* New York. W.W. Norton.

Fowler, J.W. (1981). *Stages of faith: The psychology of human development and the quest for meaning.* San Francisco: Harper and Row.

Frankl, V. (1984). *Man's search for meaning.* New York: Washington Square Press/Pocket Books.

Friedman, E.H. (1985). *Generation to generation: Family process in church and synagogue.* New York: The Guilford Press.

Gale Group (April 2000). Advice for the patient: Drug information in lay language, Buspirone (Systemic). *USP DI* [online], 1. Available online at: <http.//web7.infotrac. galegroup.com/itw/in 0_A62517785andbkm_3_1?sw_aep=uphoenixcustom>.

Gorman, J.M., Fyer, M.R., Liebowitz, M.R., and Klein, D.F. (1987). Pharmacologic provocation of panic attacks. In H.Y. Meltzer (Ed.), *Psychopharmacology: A third generation of progress* (pp. 985-993). New York: Raven Press.

Griez, E. and Schruers, K. (1998). Experimental pathophysiology of panic. *Journal of Psychosomatic Research, 45,* 493-503.

Harris, T. (1969). *I'm OK, you're OK: A practical guide to transactional analysis.* New York: Harper and Row.

Haugk, K.C. (1984). *Christian caregiving.* Minneapolis: Augsburg Press.

Haugk, K. C. (1985). *Christian caregiving: A way of life.* St. Louis: Augsburg Fortress Publishers.

Haugk, K. C. (1992). *Speaking the truth in love.* St. Louis: Steven Ministries.

Haugk, K. and McKay, W.J. (1994). *Leader's guide: Christian caregiving.* Minneapolis: Augsburg Press.

Heizer, R.F. and Kroeber, T. (1979). *Ishi, the last Yahi: A documentary history.* Berkeley, CA: University of California Press.

Hendricks, W.L. (1980). *A theology for children.* Nashville, TN: Broadman Press.

James, M. (1973). *Born to love: Transactional analysis in the church.* Reading, MA: Addison-Wesley.

Jansen, B. (2000). "Last of the Yahi" finally goes home. *Associated Press,* August 9.

Jung, C.G. (1936). *The concept of the collective unconscious: A lecture delivered before the Analytical Psychology Club of New York City.* October 2. New York: The Club.

Kahn, M. (1991). *Between therapist and client: The new relationship.* New York: W.H. Freeman and Company.

Kandel, E.R. (1983). From metapsychology to molecular biology: Explorations into the nature of anxiety. *American Journal of Psychiatry,* 140, 1277-1293.

Kaslow, F., Cooper, B., and Linsenberg, M. (1979). Family therapist authenticity as a key factor in outcome. *International Journal of Family Therapy,* 1, 194-199.

Keen, Sam. (1983). *The passionate life: Stages of loving.* San Francisco: Harper and Row.

Klerman, G.L., Hirschfield, R.M., Weissman, M.M., Pelicier, Y., Ballenger, J.C., Costa e Silva, J.A., Judd, L.L., and Keller, M.B. (Eds.) (1993). *Panic anxiety and its treatments.* Washington, DC: American Psychiatric Press.

Knox, S., Hess, S.A., Peterson, D.A., and Hill, C.E. (1997). A qualitative analysis of client perceptions of the effects of helpful therapist self-disclosure in long-term therapy. *Journal of Counseling Psychology,* 44 (3), 274-283.

Langford, D. L. (1994). Grace in an unexpected place. *Decision,* 35(2), p. 32.

Last, C., Barlow, D., and O'Brien, C. (1984). Precipitants of agoraphobia: Role of stressful life events. *Psychology Report,* 54, 567-570.

Lewis, C. S. (1960). *The four loves.* London: Geoffery Brothers.

Liege, P. A. (1965). *Consider Christian maturity.* Chicago: Priory Press.

Linn, D. and Linn, M. (1977). *Healing life's hurts: Healing memories through the five stages of forgiveness.* New York: The Paulist Press.

Loeb, S. and Ofner, A. (Eds.) (1995). *Nursing 95 drug handbook.* Springhouse, PA: Springhouse Corporation.

Maes, D. (2000). An oral interview on the subject of middle school students and systems theory. October 16.

Marney, C. (1979). *The recovery of the person.* Nashville: Abingdon.

Maslow, A. (1969). *Toward a psychology of being.* New York: Van Nostrand Reinhold.

Maslow, A. (1971). *The farther reaches of human nature.* New York: Viking Press.

May, G. (1982). *Care of mind, care of spirit: Psychiatric dimensions of spiritual direction.* San Francisco: Harper and Row.

McConnell, T.A. (1970). *The shattered self: The psychological and religious search for selfhood.* Philadelphia: The Pilgrim Press.

Medscape (2000). Empirically supported psychological treatment of panic disorder and agoraphobia. *Psychiatry and Mental Health Clinical Management,* 1, Available online at: <http://www.medscape.com/medscape/psychiatry/ClinicalMgmt/CM.v01/CMv01-04.html>.

Menninger, K. (1973). *Whatever became of sin?* New York: Hawthorne Books.

Mental Health: Facts about panic disorder (1999). drkoop.com [online]. Available online at: <wysiwyg://106/http://www.drkoop.com/dyncon/article.asp?ptp=true&id=7061&at=>.

Merton, T. (1948; copyright renewed in 1976). *The seven storey mountain.* New York: Harcourt Brace Jovanovich.

Meyers, D.G. (1978). *The human puzzle: Psychological research and Christian belief.* San Francisco: Harper and Row.

Middleton-Motz, J. (1989). *Children of trauma: Rediscovering the discarded self.* Deerfield Beach, FL: Health Communications.

Miller, A. (1981). *The drama of the gifted child.* New York: Basic Books.

Miller, A. (1988). *The untouched key: Tracing childhood trauma in creativity and destructiveness.* New York: Doubleday.

Miller, A. (1991). *Breaking down walls of silence: The liberating experience of facing painful truth.* New York: Dutton.

Miller, A. (1998). *Paths of life: Seven scenarios.* New York: Pantheon Books.

Miller, K. (1991). *Hunger for healing: The twelve steps as a classic model for Christian spiritual growth.* San Francisco: Harper.

Minirth, F.B. and Meier, P.D. (1978). *Happiness is a choice: A manual of symptoms, causes, and cures of depression.* Grand Rapids: Baker Books.

Missildine, H. (1963). *Your inner child of the past.* New York: Simon and Schuster.

Moeller, F.G. (1999). Serotonin. In *Microsoft Encarta Encyclopedia 99* (pp. 1-2). [CD-ROM]. (1993-1998). Microsoft Corporation.

Montague, G.T. (1964). *Maturing in Christ: St. Paul's program for Christian maturity.* Milwaukee, WI: Bruce Publishing Co.

Moran, G. (1979). *Education toward adulthood.* New York: Paulist Press.

Morris, L. (1981). *Testaments of love: A study of love in the Bible.* Grand Rapids, MI: Eerdmans.

Murren, D. (1999). *Churches that heal: Becoming a church that mends broken hearts and restores shattered lives.* West Monroe, LA: Howard Publishing Co.

Native American proverbs (2000). Available online at: <http://members.tripod.com/~LadySNO/NativeAmerican.html?>.

Newman, R.J., Nivat, A., and Strobel, W. (2000). Desperate hours at sea. *U.S. News and World Report,* August 28, p. 30.

Northridge, W.L. (1961). *Disorders of the emotional and spiritual life.* Great Neck, NY: Channel Press.

Norton, G.R., Pidlubny, S.R., and Norton, P.J. (1999). Prediction of panic attacks and related variables. *Behavior Therapy,* 30, 319-330.

Nouwen, H.J.M. (1969). *Intimacy.* Notre Dame, IN: Fides Publishers.

Nouwen, H.J.M. (1970). *The wounded healer.* Garden City, NY: Doubleday.

Nouwen, H.J.M. (1975). *Reaching out: The three movements of spiritual life.* Garden City, NY: Doubleday.

Oden, T.C. (1974). *Game free: The meaning of intimacy.* New York: Delta Books.

The Oxford English dictionary, Second edition. (2001).

Padovani, M.H. (1987). *Healing wounded emotions, overcoming life's hurts.* New York: Twenty Third Publications.

Peace, R. (1968). *Learning to love God . . . people . . . ourselves* (Three volumes). Downers Grove, IL: InterVarsity Press.

Peck, M.S. (1978). *The road less traveled: A new psychology of love, traditional values and spiritual growth.* New York: Simon and Schuster.

Peck, M.S. (1991). *A bed by the window.* New York: Bantam.

Peck, M.S. (1993). *A world waiting to be born: Civility rediscovered.* New York: Bantam Books.

Peck, M.S. (1995). *In search of stones: A pilgrimage of faith, reason, and discovery.* New York: Hyperion.

Pitts, F.N. and McClure, J.N. (1967). Lactate metabolism in anxiety neurosis. *New England Journal of Medicine,* 277, 1329-1336.

Powell, J. (1969). *Why am I afraid to tell you who I am?* Chicago: Argus.

Powell, J. (1976). *Fully human, fully alive: A new life through a new vision.* Allen, TX: Thomas More.

Powell, J. (1978). *Unconditional love.* Allen, TX: Argus.

Powell, J. (1984). *The Christian vision: The truth that sets us free.* Allen, TX: Argus.

Riesman, D., Glazer, N., and Denney, R. (1961). *The lonely crowd.* New Haven, CT and London: Yale University Press.

Rogers, C. (1961). *On becoming a person: A therapist's view of psychotherapy.* Boston: Houghton Mifflin Co.

Rood, W. (1972). *On nurturing Christians.* Nashville: Abingdon.

Roy-Byrne, P., Geraci, M., and Uhde, T. (1986). Life events and the onset of panic disorder. *American Journal of Psychiatry,* 143(11), 1424-1427.

Sapolsky, R.M. (1994). *Why zebras don't get ulcers: A guide to stress, stress-related diseases, and coping.* New York: W.H. Freeman.

Scanlan, M. (1974). *Inner healing.* New York: Paulist Press.

Schaef, A.W. (1990). *Escape from intimacy: The pseudo-relationship addictions.* San Francisco: Harper.

Schaef, A.W. (1992). *Beyond therapy, beyond science: A new model for healing the whole person.* San Francisco: Harper.

Schaef, A.W. (1998). *Living in process: Basic truths for living the path of the soul.* New York: Ballantine.

Schuller, R. (1982). *Self-esteem: The new reformation.* Waco, TX: Word Books.

Seamands, D.A. (1981). *Healing for damaged emotions.* Wheaton, IL: Victor Books.

Seamands, D.A. (1982). *Putting away childish things*. Wheaton, IL: Victor Books.

Seamands, D.A. (1985). *Healing of memories*. Wheaton, IL: Victor Books.

Serendipity Bible: New International Version, Tenth edition (1996). Grand Rapids, MI: Zondervan.

Seskin, S. and Shamblin, A. (1998). *Don't laugh at me* [Musical score]. Sony/ATV Tunes LLC.

Sharf, R. (1999) Psychotherapy. In *Microsoft Encarta Encyclopedia 99* (pp. 1-37). [CD-ROM]. (1993-1998). Microsoft Corporation.

Shear, M.K., Pilkonis, P.A., Cloitre, M., and Leon. A.C. (1994). Cognitive behavioral treatment compared with non-prescriptive treatment of panic disorder. *Archives of General Psychiatry*, 51, 395-401.

Simon, J.C. (1988). Criteria for therapist self-disclosure. *American Journal of Psychotherapy*, 42, 404-415.

Simons, J. and Reidy, J. (1968). *The trick of loving*. New York: Herder and Herder.

Stein, M.B., Jang, K.L., and Livesley, J.W. (1999). Heritability of anxiety sensitivity: A twin study. *The American Journal of Psychiatry*, 156 (February), 246-251.

Steiner, C.E. (1974). *Scripts people live: Transactional analysis and life scripts*. New York: Bantam Books.

Stokes, K. (Ed.) (1981). *Faith development in the adult life cycle*. New York: W.H. Sadler.

Stone, H. (1991). *The caring church: A guide for lay pastoral care*. Philadelphia: Fortress Press.

Strunk, O. Jr. (1965). *Mature religion: A psychological study*. Nashville: Abingdon.

Tanner, I.J. (1965). *Loneliness: The fear of love: An application of transactional analysis*. San Francisco: Harper and Row.

Teilhard de Chardin, P. (1972). *On love*. London: Collins.

Torgersen, S. (1990). Twin studies in panic disorder. In J.C. Ballenger (Ed.), *Neurobiology of panic disorder*, Volume 6: *Frontiers of clinical neuroscience* (pp. 51-58). New York: Wiley-Liss.

Tournier, P. (1957). *The meaning of persons*. New York: Harper and Row.

Tournier, P. (1962). *Escape from loneliness*. Philadelphia: Westminster.

Tournier, P. (1962). *Grace and guilt*. New York: Harper and Row.

Tournier, P. (1963). *The strong and the weak*. Philadelphia: Westminster.

Tournier, P. (1964). *The whole person in a broken world*. New York: Harper and Row.

Tournier, P. (1965). *Healing of persons*. New York: Harper and Row.

Tournier, P. (1966). *The person reborn*. New York: Harper and Row.

Tournier, P. (1968). *A place for you: Psychology and religion*. New York: Harper and Row.

Tournier, P. (1973). *The adventure of living*. New York: Harper and Row.

Tournier, P. (1978). *The violence within*. San Francisco: Harper and Row.

Tournier, P. (1979). *The healing spirit*. Westchester, IL: Good News.

Twemlow, S.W. (1997). Exploitation of patients: Themes in the psychopathology of their therapists. *American Journal of Psychotherapy,* 51 (3), 357+. Available online at: <http://ehostvgw2.epnet.com/delivery.asp?d...nts&startHitNum=4&rlStartHit= 4& delType= FT>.

Twemlow, S.W. and Gabbard, G.O. (1981). Iatrogenic disease or doctor-patient collusion. *American Family Physician,* 24, 129-134.

von Bertalanffy, L. (1974). General system theory and psychiatry. In A. Silvano (Ed.), *American handbook of psychiatry,* Volume 1 (pp. 1095-1117). New York: Basic Books, Inc.

Wachtel, P.L. (1993). *Therapeutic communication: Principles and effective practice.* New York: The Guilford Press.

Ware, F.R. (1962). *Psychological concepts of maturing.* Philadelphia: AAAS Symposium.

Warters, J. (1949). *Achieving maturity.* New York: McGraw-Hill.

Weeks, L.B. (1999). John Calvin. In *Microsoft Encarta Encyclopedia 99* (pp. 1-5). [CD-ROM]. (1993-1998). Microsoft Corporation.

Weiss, S.R. and Uhde, T.W. (1990). Animal models of anxiety. In J.C. Ballenger (Ed.), *Neurobiology of panic disorder,* Volume 8: *Frontiers of clinical neuroscience* (pp. 3-27). New York: Wiley-Liss.

Westerhoff, J.H. (1979). *Inner growth, outer change: An educational guide to church renewal.* New York: Seabury Press.

What are the current treatments for panic disorder? (2000, May). *The Harvard Mental Health Letter,* 16(11) Available online at: <http://ehostvgw7.epnet.com/ delivery.asp?d...der&startHitNum=1&rlStartHit=1&delType=FT>.

Whitfield, C. (1989). *Healing the child within: Discovery and recovery for adult children of dysfunctional families.* Deerfield Beach, FL: Health Communications.

Whitfield, C. (1990). *A gift to myself: A personal workbook and guide to healing my child within.* Deerfield Beach, FL: Health Communications.

Whitfield, C. and Amodeo, J. (1993). *Boundaries and relationships: Knowing, protecting and enjoying the self.* Deerfield Beach, FL: Health Communications.

Woolman, S. and Brown, M. (1979). *T.A.: The total handbook of transactional analysis.* Englewood Cliffs, NJ: Prentice-Hall.

Wright, N. (1985). *Making peace with your past.* Old Tappan, NJ: Revell.

Young, R. (1982). *Young's analytical concordance to the Bible* (Revision of the 1881 edition). Nashville, TN: Thomas Nelson Publishers.

Index

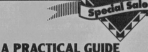

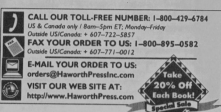